Man and His Foods

Man and His Foods

Studies in the Ethnobotany of Nutrition-Contemporary, Primitive, and Prehistoric Non-European Diets

Papers Presented at the Eleventh International Botanical Congress

(Seattle, Washington)
(August 24–September 2, 1969)

General Editor
C. Earle Smith, Jr.

THE UNIVERSITY OF ALABAMA PRESS
University, Alabama

ISBN 0-8173-2400-3
Library of Congress Number Card Catalog 77-38705

Manufactured in the United States of America

Contents

Contributors

Jacques Barrau, Assistant Director, Laboratoire d'Ethnobotanique, Museum Nacional d'Histoire Naturelle de Paris, France

Eric O. Callen,* Professor of Plant Pathology, McGill University, Quebec, Canada

Lawrence Kaplan, Professor of Biology, University of Massachusetts, Boston, Massachusetts

N. H. Nickerson, Professor of Biology, Tufts University, Medford, Massachusetts 02155

E. A. Richter, U.S. Public Health Service, Lame Deer, Montana

N. H. Rowe, Professor of Oral Pathology, School of Dentistry, University of Michigan, Ann Arbor, Michigan 48104

C. Earle Smith, Jr., Professor of Anthropology and Biology, University of Alabama, Tuscaloosa, Alabama (previously, New Crops Research Branch, Agricultural Research Service, USDA, Beltsville, Maryland)

Aubrey W. Williams, Jr., Professor of Anthropology, University of Maryland, College Park, Maryland 20742

*deceased

Introduction

C. Earle Smith, Jr.

Ethnobotany of Nutrition is the germ of a concept that must play an ever increasing role in the interpretation of man's existence. We are all vitally aware of the impending population crisis as it is seen in the light of today's dietary levels among peoples of north European extraction. We are also aware of the famines that have periodically beset the people of parts of Asia. But, how much do we truly know about the nutrition of human beings who do not eat the diet common among peoples of European extraction?

Our symposium title is broad enough to cover approaches from many different angles. Certainly not the least important of these approaches is the chemistry of foods utilized by non-Europeans. An exact account of the nutritional balance of widely differing diets could have occupied the entire symposium timetable. Unfortunately, the food chemists and nutritionists were unable to meet with us at this XI International Botanical Congress. Therefore, I assembled as broad a summary of the nutrition of non-European peoples as could be encompassed within the short time available for the symposium.

The contributors have amply fulfilled their roles in approaching this goal. For the first time, the outlines of nutritional patterns for a single area are considered, from early hunting-gathering people to today's population in Mexico in presentations by Eric O. Callen and Aubrey W. Williams. Norton H. Nickerson, N. H. Rowe, and E. A. Richter provide evidence for a previously unreported abundance of plant foods in the diets of Eskimo populations on the North slope of Alaska. A totally different nutritional pattern is summarized by Jacques Barrau for the peoples of the Pacific islands. A single nutritional source, beans in the Mesoamerican diet, is considered by Lawrence Kaplan from the standpoint of complementary amino acids.

These papers provide few final answers. Information on the nutritional level of unusual diets is currently unavailable. For the most part, ethnobotany has been concerned with reporting the use of cultivated and gathered native plants as food. Nutritional analyses showing the amount of available minerals, proteins, and carbohydrates have been published for foods collected in Latin America, Africa, and elsewhere, but few attempts have been made to assess the daily nutritional intake of a family or the people of a village using a non-European diet. Only after these data are gathered can we begin to find answers to many nutritional problems. It is hoped that studies will be undertaken which will eventually lead to an understanding of the energy cycles involved in local nutritional patterns. We may then begin to think in terms of repatterning nutritional intake for a more efficient use of the world's food supply.

One of the enigmas which Williams' paper suggests is the vigor and activity of people who use substantially lower amounts of calories than we are accustomed to regard as essential. Callen's data suggest that this pattern was not essentially different in the past in Mexico, yet the early Mexicans built prodigious architectural monuments under what must have been a complex social system. People on the verge of starvation could not have accomplished so much. Perhaps we will find differing patterns in human basal metabolism which enable some peoples to make more efficient use of their caloric intake.

Nickerson explains the intake of vitamins and minerals in the diets of Eskimos who were thought to have subsisted largely on animal foods. The ingenious use of a preserving technique provides these Eskimos with access to plant foods, and therefore vitamins, throughout the long winter of the northern latitudes.

Barrau summarizes unusual movement of subsistence foods across the vast reaches of the Pacific Ocean. Unlike the previous authors who deal with nutritional patterns developed from plants in the native flora, Barrau finds that the peoples from New Guinea through Polynesia have carried with them the basic tuberous food plants as well as the ancient agricultural practices originated by their ancestors in tropical southeast Asia. He suggests that disturbance of the old pattern has caused more nutritional deficiency than was normal when the traditional cultivates were the sole basis for the diet. Detailed nutritional data are woefully lacking for individuals and villages in Oceania.

A look at the complementary roles of amino acids from beans and corn allows Kaplan to raise many interesting speculations regarding mechanisms controlling the selection of complementary varieties of beans and the historical pattern of protein source replacement in Mesoamerica. In spite of the more sophisticated data available for beans, many questions must remain unanswered pending more concentrated study.

To sum up, our contributors present a nucleus for the ethnobotanical study of nutrition. Their facts perhaps show the gaps in our knowledge more clearly than they summarize the total knowledge available to us. The only logical solution is apparent. A totally new field, ethnobotany of nutrition, staffed by scientists skilled in both the broad fellowship tactics of ethnology and the detailed skills of the nutritional chemist, must be created to collect the data to fill the gaps in knowledge. Until this unstudied field of knowledge has been tilled, we cannot hope to reap a harvest to allay the world's nutritional problems.

Inherent in this pioneering effort is both a warning and a threat. Almost complete lack of understanding of the nutritional patterns of the bulk of the world's population—those peoples that do not subsist on the standard European diet—indicates that we are doomed to failure in our efforts to gain in the race between population growth and the production of food supplies. This is the threat. Acculturation is proceeding so rapidly among smaller ethnic groups that we will soon be unable to collect data on their nutritional patterns. This is the warning. May we have sufficient wisdom to heed both.

Man and His Foods

N. H. Nickerson, N. H. Rowe, E. A. Richter

NATIVE PLANTS IN THE DIETS OF NORTH ALASKAN ESKIMOS

Tribal man, because of his dietary habits, is a reflection of the ecosystems of his area. In recent papers (Covich and Nickerson, 1966; Nickerson and Covich, 1966; Rowe and Johnson, 1964; Sexton, Heatwole, and Knight, 1964), some aspects of the ecology of Panama's Darièn province and of the Chocó Indians who dwell there have been explored and documented. As a part of the continuing studies on the relationships between the diet and the dental health of isolated human groups, similar studies were undertaken on the Amerinds referred to by Spencer and Jennings (1965) as the North Alaskan Eskimos. Because there is geographic variation in human health and disease, these situations, as Stamp (1965) has noted, afford unique opportunities both to identify etiology and further our understandings of human pathogenesis on the one

*This research was supported in part by a grant to the first author from the Tufts University Faculty Research Fund, and in part by a Public Health Service grant to the second author. The cooperation of the Arctic Research Laboratory through its director, Max Brewer, is gratefully acknowledged.

hand and, on the other, to accumulate data concerning plant uses of interest and value to ethnology and botany.

The purposes of this study, conducted in the field during the summer of 1965, were twofold: to identify incidence and severity of oral disease in the Eskimo (Rowe *et al.*, 1969), and to assess the extent to which the Arctic flora is utilized by the Eskimo as a dietary constituent. The second of these objectives is reported on here.

Utilization of native plants as common dietary items in a country locked in ice for so much of the year would seem improbable and at best unimportant, as reference to Murdoch (1892), Stoney (1899), Ford (1959) and Spencer and Jennings (1965), seemingly confirms. Yet knowledge of edible plants is apparently a part of the Eskimo ancient culture, the development of which has enabled the individual to survive in the formidable Arctic environment.

Method of Data Collection

Information about plant usage was gathered by subject interrogation. The eagerness of the Eskimo to provide answers he felt we might wish to hear originally posed a dilemma which was overcome and turned to advantage by utilizing a widely known and respected Eskimo, Pete Sovalik, as conversationalist and interpreter. His acceptance by interviewees, adeptness at questioning, and familiarity with both English and the several North Alsakan Inupiak (Eskimo) dialects added a needed dimension to the validity and comprehensiveness of our investigation.

Data were obtained at four separate sites: Koktuvik on Barter Island, Barrow Village near Point Barrow, Wainwright, and Anaktuvuk Pass. (See map, Fig. 1.) The first three sites were coastal villages; the last is located south and inland 200 miles from Barrow just into the Brooks Range.

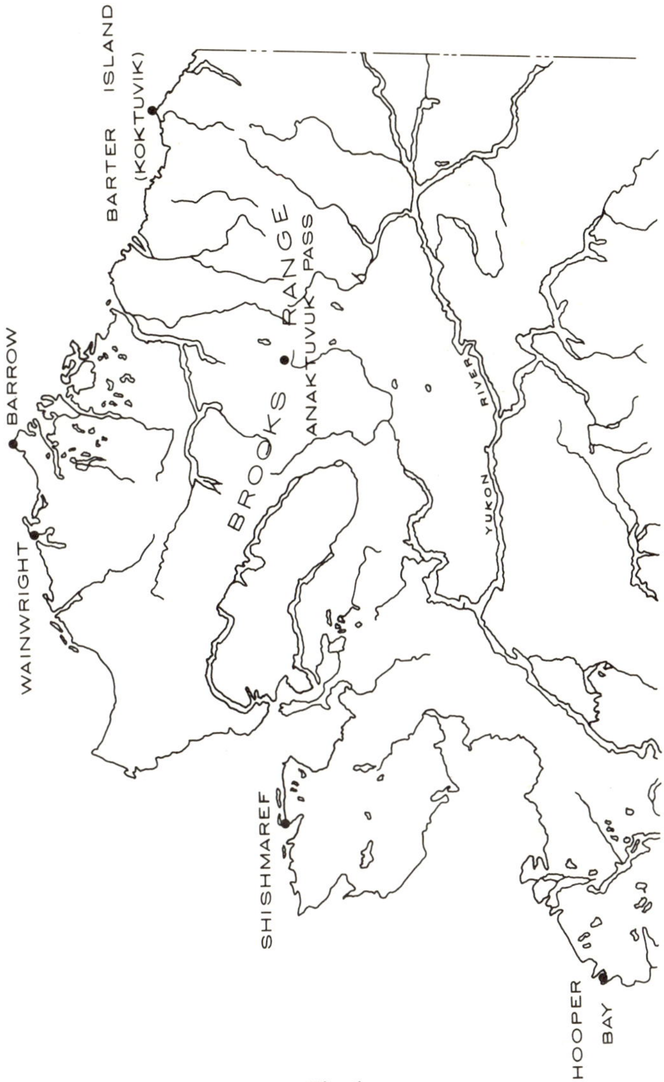

Fig. 1

Map of Alaska, showing village sites visited and areas from which plants and plant-use information have been collected.

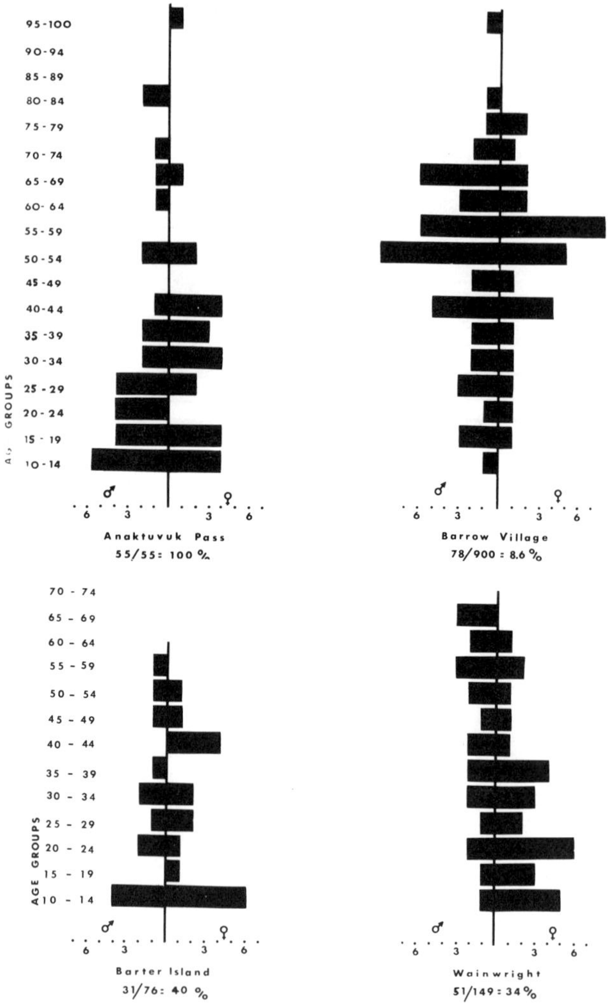

Fig. 2

Population structures of four villages on the Alaskan North Slope as determined in August, 1965. Percentages indicate fractions of total populations sampled at each site. See text for further comments.

The number of adult Eskimos interviewed approximated 9% of the population over 10 years of age at Barrow, 34% at Wainright, 41% at Barter, and 100% at Anaktuvuk Pass. Age-sex population distributions of the sites are shown in Fig. 2. The samples of less than 100% are not necessarily random, however. Barrow's interviewees, for instance, were mostly connected with the Arctic Research Laboratory. At Wainright, some 20 families were away in the interior picking berries and hunting; similarly, at Barter Island, 30 people were on a hunting and berrying expedition to the interior. Our percentages are based on local 1965 census records in every village except Barrow.

Searches were conducted and collections made on lands adjacent to each of the four village sites to verify local occurrences and provide specimens of each dietary plant. Voucher specimens are deposited in the Tufts University Herbarium; a duplicate set has been deposited in the Economic Plants Herbarium of Oakes Ames at Harvard University, Cambridge.

Observations

Several food plants were available at each of the four village sites visited, in spite of the fact that these same plants had seldom been referred to by previous investigators or, for that matter, by the Eskimos themselves (Murdoch, 1892; Spencer, 1959; Spencer and Jennings, 1965).

Table I presents the English-Eskimo plant name equivalents and their scientific names based on the works of Anderson (1959) and Wiggins and Thomas (1962), insofar as we were able to determine their identity from both our own studies and those of the others. Tables II through V present the information arranged by age of informant, with the oldest first and the youngest last, substantially as

TABLE I

Eskimo Food Plants

North Alaskan Eskimo Name (spellings from Pete Sovalik)	West Alaskan Eskimo Name (Shishmaref Cook Book)	Common English Name	Scientific Name (based on dried specimens)	Villages where collected: B - Barrow, AP - Anaktuvuk Pass, W - Wainwright, K - Koktuvik, H - Hooper Bay*				
				B	AP	W	K	H
kuagak, quagak	cahak	spinach, greens	Rumex arcticus	X	X	X	X	
ipich	nizekmeektak	wild chard	Polygonum bistorta					
kungulik		spinach	Oxyria digyna				X	
masu	mah-zee	roots	Oxytropus maydelliana	X			X	
			Oxytropus arctica					
			Oxytropus campestris		X		X	
			var. varians		X			
			Pedicularis lanata		X			
			Pedicularis sudetica					X
			Pedicularis chamissonis			X	X	
			Pedicularis langsdorfii var. arctica	X				X
okpik	seurah	willow buds	Salix					X
		shoots & leaves	Salix richardsonii					X

			Salix glacialis	X				
			Salix pulchra	X	X		X	
			Salix rotundifolia		X			
			Salix alaxensis		X	X		
			Salix glauca var. acutifolia		X		X	
			Salix phlebophylla		X	X		
			Salix arctica		X		X	
asiavik	suewuk	blueberries	Vaccinium parviflorum				X	
			Vaccinium uliginosum		X			
kipmiknak	kepmingyuk	cranberries	Vaccinium vitis-idaea		X	X	X	
paungak	ahzeeuk	blackberry	Empetrum nigrum		X		X	X
angutvak		red berry	Arctostaphylos alpina var. rubra		X			
kavlak		blackberry	Arctostaphylos alpina var. alpina		X			X
akpik	akpik	salmonberry	Rubus chamaemorus		X	X		X
kasaguak	fermented lichens from the rumen of the caribou		(A delicacy to older Eskimos, almost completely disdained by younger ones.)					X

*Hooper Bay collections made by Dr. R. T. Holmes, Dartmouth College, Hanover, N.H.

TABLE II

Anaktuvuk Pass

Case Number	Sex, Age, % Eskimo	Asiavik blueberries	Akpik salmon-berries	Kipmikuak cranberries	Paugnak black-berries	Masu roots	Kuagak dock	Okpik willow shoots, leaves	Kasaguak caribou rumen, lichens	Nuagavik white clay
A49	F-95-E	++++	++++	++++	++++	++++	++++	+++	++++	++(+)
A2	M-82-E	++++	++++	++++	++++	++++	++++	++++	+++	+++
A5	M-80-E	+++	+++	+++	+++	+++	+++	+	+++	++(+)
A31	M-71-E	+++	+++	+++	+++	+++	++	+++	++	++(+)
A13	F-69-E	+++	+++	+++	+++	+++	+++			++
A14	M-65E	+++	+++	++++	+++	+++	+++		+++	++(+)
A24	M-61-E	+++	+++	+++	+++	+++	++(+)		++	++
A15	M-53-E	+++	+++	+++	+++	+++	+++	+++		++(+)
A35	F-51-E	+++	+++	+++	+++	+++	+++		++(+)	++(+)
A11	M-50-E	+++	+++	+++	+++	+++	+++	+		++(+)
A12	F-50-E	+++	+++	+++	+++	+++		+		++(+)
A10	F-44-E	+++	+++	+++	+++	+++	+++	θ		++(+)
A32	F-44-E	+++	+++	+++	+++	+++	+++		++(+)	++(+)
A9	F-43-E	+++	+++	+++	+++	+++	+	+		++(+)
A1	M-42-E	+++	+++	+++	+++	++	+++	+++		++(+)
A23	F-40-E	+++	+++	+++	+++	+	++	++	++(+)	++
A17	F-38-E	+++	+++	+++	+++	+++	+++	+++		++
A22	M-38-E	+++	+++	+++	+++	+++	+	++(+)	++(+)	++(+)
A20	M-36-E	+++	+++	+++	+++	+	+	+		++(+)
A16	F-35-E	+++	+++	+++	+++	+++				++(+)
A19	F-35-E	+++	+++	+++	+++	+++	+	+		++(+)
A8	F-34-E	++++	++++	++++	++++	++++	+++	+++		++(+)

A33	F-32-E	+++	+++	+++	+++	+++	+++		++(+)	++(+)
A21	F-31-E	+++	+++	+++	+++	+++	+	+		0
A6	M-30-E	++(+)	++(+)	++(+)	++(+)	+		+		++
A48	M-32-E	++	++	++	++	++	+	++	+	0
A50	F-30-E								++(+)	++(+)
A4	M-29-E	+++	+++	+++	+++	++	+	+	+	+
A34	F-29-E	+++	+++	+++	+++	+++	+++	++(+)	+++	++(+)
A53	M-27-E	+++	+++	+++	+++	+++	+	+		+
A57	M-27-E	+++	+++	+++	+++	+++		+++	0	0
A7	M-25-E	+++	+++	+++	+++	+++	+			+
A51	F-25-E	+++	+++	+++	+	+	+++		+	0
A40	M-23-E	+++	+++	+++	+++	+++	++(+)	+++	+	0
A3	M-21-E	+++	+++	+++	+++	+	+	+		+
A41	M-20-E	+++	+++	+++	+++	+++	+	+++	+	0
A54	M-20-E	+++	+++	+++	+++	+	+	+	0	++
A52	M-19-E	+++	+++	+++	+++	+	+	+++	0	0
A18	F-18-E	+++	+++	+++	+++	+++	+++	+++		0
A28	F-17-E	+++	+++	+++	+++				+	+
A55	M-17-E	+++	+++	+++	+++	+++	+	+++	+	+
A27	F-16-E	+++	+++	+++	+++				+	+
A29	M-16-E	+++	+++	+++	+++				0	0
A26	F-15-E	+++	+++	+++	+++		+			+
A56	M-15-E	+++	+++	+++	+++	+	+	+	+	0
A39	M-14-E	+++	+++	+++	+++	++	+	++	+	0
A30	M-14-E	+++	+++	+++	+++	++	++	++	+	+
A38	M-14-E	+++	+++	+++	+++	+	++	+	+	0
A25	M-13-E	+++	+++	+++	+++			+		

TABLE III

Barrow Village

Case Number	Sex, Age, % Eskimo	Asiavik blueberries	Akpik salmon-berries	Kipmikuak cranberries	Paugnak black-berries	Maso roots	Kuagak dock	Okpik willow shoots, leaves	Kasaguak caribou rumen, lichens	Nuagavik white clay
31	M-100-E	++++	++++	++++	++++	++++	++++	++++	++++	+++
13	M-80-E	++++	++++	++++	++++	++++	++++	++++	++++	+++
53	F-77-E	++++	++++	++++	++++		++++	++++		+
42	M-76-E	+++	+++	+++	+++	+++	+++	+++		+++
2	F-75-7/8-E	+++	+++	+++	+++	+++	+++	+++		+++
36	M-74-E	+++	+++	+++	+++	+++				+++
58	F-74-E	+++	+++	+++	+++	++(+)	++(+)	+		++
32	M-72-½E	+++	+++	+++	+++					++
41	F-69-E	++++	++++	++++	++++	+++	+++			+
39	M-67-E	+++	+++	+++	+++		+++	+++		+
37	F-67-E	+++	+++	+++	+++	+++	+++	+++	+	0
28	F-67-E	+++	+++	+++	+++			+		0
6	M-67-E	+++	+++	+++	+++				+++	
25	M-66-E	+++	+++	+++	+++					++(+)
57	F-65-E	++++	++++	++++	++++	+++	+	+		+++
59	M-65-E	++++	++++	++++	++++	+++	+	+++		+++
35	M-65-E	++++	++++	++++	++++			+		+
15	M-64-½E	++++	++++	++++	++++		+++	+++		
8	M-62-E	++++	++++	++++	++++	++++	+++	++++	++++	+++
5	M-62-7/8E	++++	++++	++++	++++	++++	+++	++++	++++	+++
16	F-62-E	+++	+++	+++	+++	+++	+++	+		
30	F-59-E	+++	+++	+++	+++	++++	+++	+++		+

75	M-58-E	+++	+++	+++	+++	+	+++	+++	+++	0
65	M-58-E	+++	+++	+	+	+++	+++	+	+++	0
23	F-58-E	+++	+++	+++	+++	++++	+++	+++		
27	F-58-E	+++	+++	+++	+++	+++	+++	+++		0
33	M-58-E	+++	+++	+++	+++	+++	+++	+++		+
20	M-57-E	++++	++++	++++	++++	+++	+++	+++		++(+)
45	F-57-E	+++	+++	+++	+++	+++	+++	+++	+++	+
29	F-56-E	+++	+++	+++	+++	+++	+++	+++		0
70	M-56-E	+++	+++	+	+++	+++	+++	+	+++	+
24	F-56-3/4E	+++	+++	+++	+++	+++	+++	+++		+
17	F-55-3/4E	+	+	++++	++++					
3	F-55-E	+	+	+	+	+	+	+	+	
68	M-55-E	+	+++	+	+++	+	+	+	+++	0
78	M-54-E	+	+	+	+	+	+	+	+++	++
4	M-53-E	+++	+	+++	+					
10	F-53-E	+++	+++	+++	+++	+++		+++		
12	F-53-E						+++			
34	M-53-E	+++	+++	+++	+++					+
67	M-52-E	+++	+++	+++	+++	+	+++	+	+++	0
77	M-51-E	++(+)	++(+)	++(+)	++(+)	++(+)	++(+)	++(+)	+++	++
1	M-51-E	++++	++(+)	++(+)	++(+)					
11	F-51-E	+++	+++	+++	+++	+				
19	F-51-3/4E	+++	+++	+++	+++	+	+++	+++		+
38	M-51-E	+++	+++	+++	+++					0
74	M-50-3/4E	+++	+	+	+	+++	+++	+	+++	++
7	F-50-E	+	+	+	+			+++		
18	M-50-E	+++	+++	+++	+++	+++	+++	+++		++
61	M-49-E	+++	+++	+++	+++	+++	+++	+++		++
48	M-46-3/4E	++	++	++	++	++	++	++	++	+
9	F-45-3/4E	+++	+++	+++	+++			+++		

table III cont

Case Number	Sex, Age, % Eskimo	Asiavik blueberries	Akpik salmon-berries	Kipmikuak cranberries	Paugnak black-berries	Maso roots	Kuagak dock	Okpik willow shoots, leaves	Kasaguak caribou rumen, lichens	Nuagavik white clay
56	F-44-E	+++	+++	+++	+++	+	+++	+		+
63	M-44-E	+++	+++	+++	+++	+++	+++	+++	+++	0
52	F-43-3/4E	+	+	+	+	+	+++			+
44	M-43-E	+++	+++	+++	+++					0
46	F-43-E									
64	M-42-E	++	++	++	++	++	++	++	+++	+
72	M-40-E	+++	+++	+++	+++	+++	+++	+++	+++	+
73	M-40-E	++	++	++	++	+	+	+++	+	0
47	F-40-E	+++	+++	+++	+++	+++	+++	+		++(+)
71	M-39-E	+++	+++	+++	+++	+++	+++	+++	+++	++
40	F-38-E	++++	++++	++++	++++	+++				
49	M-36-E									
14	F-33-E	++++	++++	++++	++++	+++	+++	+++		
69	M-31-E	+++	+++	+++	+++	+	+++	+++	+++	+
66	M-30-E	+++	+++	+++	+++	+	+++	+++	+++	0
54	M-29-E	+++	+++	+++	+++	+++	+++	+		+
26	M-28-E	+	+	+	+	+	+	+	+++	
55	F-27-E	+++	+++	+++	+++	+	+++	+		+
62	M-25-E	+++				+++	+++	+++		
43	F-24-E	+	+++	+++	+	+++	+	+	+	+
76	M-28-7/8E	+++	+++	+	+++	+++	+++	+++	+	0
51	M-19-E	++	++	++	++	+	+	+	+	+
50	M-18-E									
60	F-16-E	++	++	++	++	++	++	++		+
21	M-15/16E	+	+	+	+	+	+	+	++	+
22	M-14-E									

it was obtained from each village. Table VI explains the symbols used under each of the Eskimo plant names.

The first column of Tables II through V is the number of the order of interviewing which occurred. The second column, headed "Code," gives in order the sex, age, and percentage of Eskimo blood. A single "E" means a full-blooded Eskimo, 1/2E means half-Eskimo, and so on. Interestingly, shovel-shaped incisors, a genetic trait found routinely among the Chocó in Darièn, also appear in the North Alaskan Eskimo. The trait is so easily noted that the degree of its presence or absence is a close indicator of the percentage of Eskimo blood in the examinee. We verified this by questioning other members of the community as well as the subject himself.

The use of caribou stomach (rumen) contents as a highly prized food was described to us by many older individuals and by Mr. Sovalik. The food material consists mostly of lichens, and is not "moss," as Murdoch (1892) and Spencer and Jennings (1965) called it. It is fermented in the excised rumen for 2 or 3 days prior to its consumption.

A curious reference to "white, edible, sweet clay," first found in Stoney (1899), and the possibility of its role in Eskimo dental health, led us to ask each informant about the use of this clay. Its recognition and use are more than casual, but white clay was not a common and consistent part of the diet in any location.

Berries, roots, and greens of several kinds are routinely eaten fresh. Berries are often mixed with oogruk (bearded seal) oil and stored in sealskin bags in the family freezer room, a 10- to 12-foot-deep hole into the permafrost, complete with ladder, which is kept closed by skins or canvas.

The North Alaskan Eskimo has not domesticated any

TABLE IV

Koktuvik
(Barter Island)

Case Number	Sex, Age, % Eskimo	Asiavik blueberries	Akpik salmon-berries	Kipmikuak cranberries	Paugnak black-berries	Maso roots	Kuagak dock	Okpik willow shoots, leaves	Kasaguak caribou rumen, lichens	Nuagavik white clay
K28	M-56-E	++	++	++	++	++(+)	++(+)	++(+)	++(+)	0
K23	F-53-½E	++(+)	++(+)	++(+)	++(+)	+++	+++	θ	++	0
K29	M-51-E	++(+)	++(+)	++(+)	++(+)	++(+)	+	+++	+++	0
K8	M-48-3/4E	++(+)	++(+)	++(+)	++(+)	++(+)	++(+)	++(+)	++(+)	0
K19	F-45-E	+++	+++	+++	+++	++(+)	++(+)	++(+)	+++	+
K5	F-44-E	++(+)	++(+)	++(+)	++(+)	++(+)	++(+)	++(+)	++(+)	0
K7	F-43-3/4E									
K31	F-42-E	++(+)	++++	++(+)	++(+)	++++	++(+)	++(+)	++++	0
K24	F-40-E	++(+)	++++	++(+)	++(+)	+++	+++	+	+++	0
K3	M-36-3/4E	+++	+++	+++	+++	+	+	+	+	0
K6	F-34-3/4E	++(+)	++(+)	++(+)	++(+)	++	+	+++	+	0
K27	M-33-E	++(+)	++(+)	++(+)	++(+)	+	+	+	+++	0

K20	F -32-3/4E	++(+)	++(+)	++(+)	++(+)	++(+)	++(+)	++(+)	+	0
K2	M-32-E	++(+)	++(+)	++(+)	++(+)	++(+)	++(+)	++(+)	++(+)	
K10	F -26-3/4E	+	+	+	+	+	+++	+	+	+
K25	M-25-E	+	+	+	+	+	++	++	+	0
K30	F -25-3/4E	+	+	+	+	+	+	+	+	0
K26	F -24-E	+++	+++	+++	+++	+	+	+	+	0
K1	M-21-3/4E	++(+)	++(+)	++(+)	++(+)	++(+)	++(+)	++(+)	+	0
K16	M-20-E	+++	+	+	+	+	+	+	0	0
K17	F -16-7/8E	++(+)	++(+)	++(+)	++(+)	+	+	+	0	0
K9	F -14-E	+	+	+	+	+	+	+	+++	0
K14	M-14-E	+	+	+	+	0	0	0	++	0
K15	M-14-7/8E	0	0	0	0	0	0	0	0	0
K18	F -13-3/4E	0	0	0	0	0	0	0	0	0
K4	M-13-3/4E	+++	+++	+++	+++	+	+	+++	+	0
K13	M-13-E	+++	+++	+++	+++	0	0	0	0	0
K11	F -12-E	0	0	0	0	0	0	0	0	+
K12	F 12-E	++	++	++	++	0	0	0	++	0
K21	F -11-E	0	0	0	0	0	0	0	0	0
K22	F -11-E	0	0	0	0	0	0	0	0	0

TABLE V

Wainwright

Case Number	Sex, Age, % Eskimo	Asiavik blueberries	Akpik salmon-berries	Kipmikuak cranberries	Paugnak black-berries	Maso roots	Kuagak dock	Okpik willow shoots, leaves	Kasaguak caribou rumen, lichens	Naugavik white clay
W11	M-68-E	+++	+++	+++	+++	+++	+++	+++	+++	++(+)
W46	M-67-E	+++	+++	+++	+++	++(+)	+++	++(+)	+++	+
W43	M-66-E	++(+)	++(+)	++(+)	++(+)	++(+)	++(+)	++(+)	+++	++
W36	M-63-E	++(+)	++(+)	++(+)	++(+)	+	+++	+	+++	++(+)
W2	F-62-E	+	+++	+	+	+	+	+	++	+
W24	M-61-½E	+++	+++	+++	+++	+++	+++	+++	+++	+++
W51	M-57-E	+++	+++	+++	+++	+	+++	+++	+++	+
W12	M-570½E	+++	+++	+++	+++	+	+	+++	+	+
W5	M-57-E	+++	+++	+++	+++	+++	+++	+++	+++	0
W52	F-56-E	++(+)	++(+)	++(+)	++(+)	+	+++	+++	+++	0
W48	F-55-E	+	+	+	+	+	+++	+		+
W13	M-53-E	++(+)	++(+)	++(+)	++(+)	++(+)	++(+)	++(+)		
W49	F-53-E	++	++	++	++	++	+++	++	+++	++(+)
W25	M-50-E	++	++	++	++	++	+++	++	+++	
W6	F-48-E	+++	+++	+++	+++	++	++	++	0	0
W38	M-48-E	++(+)	++(+)	++(+)	++(+)	++(+)	+++	+++	+++	+
W50	M-47-E	+++	+++	+++	+++	+	+	+	+++	0
W40	M-43-E	+++	+++	+++	+++	+	+++	+	+++	0
W41	F-41-E	+	+	+	+	+	+	+	++	0
W1	M-38-3/4E	+	+	+	+	+	+	++(+)	+	+
W3	F-37-E	++	++	++	++	+	+++	+++	0	0
W4	F-37-3/4E	+++	+++	+++	+++	+	+++	+++	+	+
W8	F-36-E	++	++	++	++	+++	+++	+	+++	0
W20	F-36-E	+	+++	+	+	+	+	+	+	0

W42	M-35-E	+	+	+	+	+	+	+	+	0
W47	F-34-E	+	+	+	+	+	+	+	+++	0
W39	M-32-E	+++	+++	+++	+++	+++	+++	+++	+++	+
W44	M-31-E	++(+)	++(+)	++(+)	++(+)	++	+	+	+	0
W9	F-31-E									
W28	F-30-E	+++	++++	+++	+++	+	+++	+	+++	0
W16	F-26-E	+	+	+	+	+	++	+	++	0
W7	M-26-E	++	++	++	++	++	++	++	++	0
W15	F-25-E	+	+	+	+	+	+	++	+	0
W29	F-24-E	+++	+++	+++	+++	+	+	+	+++	0
W17	F-24-E	+	+	+	+	+	+	+	+	0
W26	F-22-E	+	+	+	+	+	+++	+	+	0
W32	M-21-E	++++	++++	++++	++++	+	++	++	+++	+
W33	M-21-E	++	++	++	++	+	++	+	+	0
W35	F-21-E	+	+	+	+	+	+++	+	+	0
W27	F-21-E	++	++	++	++	++	+++	+++	+++	0
W10	F-20-E									
W37	F-19-E	0	0	0	0	0	0	0	0	0
W19	F-18-E	0	0	0	0	0	0	0	0	0
W34	F-18-E	0	0	0	0	0	+++	0	0	0
W14	M-17-E	++	++	++	++	++	++	+++	0	0
W21	M-14-E	0	+++	0	0	0	++	0	+++	0
W30	F-14-E	0	0	0	0	0	+++	0	0	0
W22	F-13-E	0	0	0	++	0	0	0	+++	0
W31	F-12-7/8E	0	0	0	0	0	+++	+++	0	0
W18	F-12-E	++	++	++	++	0	0	0	0	0
W45	F-10-E									

TABLE VI

KEY TO SYMBOLS USED IN TABLES II - V

0	never heard of item
+	heard of item
++	tried item
++(+)	used item when young (in past)
+++	used item regularly in season
++++	item stored for off-season use
⊕	parents used item; individual does not use item now
Blank	no information available

plant as a crop in the sense of giving it horticultural care, yet plants and their uses are well-known, especially among older inhabitants and in the inland village of Anaktuvuk Pass. Roots (masu) of several species of *Pedicularis* and *Oxytropis* are eaten fresh or boiled. Young willow shoots (okpik) are eaten green, either as harvested or dipped in oogruk oil. Leaves and herbaceous stems of *Oxyria, Rumex,* and *Polygonum,* are variously called spinach, greens, or wild chard (kuagak, kungulik, ipich). They are most often boiled before being eaten. Fish may be cooked in the same pot, and the whole eaten as a stew. On occasion, fresh greens may be finely cut, mixed with oogruk oil, and consumed as a salad, especially by women and children. Greens are generally eaten only in season because the growth is relatively tender.

The major dietary item of the Anaktuvuk Pass dwellers is caribou meat. It is most often eaten in the fresh-frozen state or aged-frozen state (kwak), and forms the bulk of each of the three daily meals. Oogruk oil, sometimes with blueberries or cranberries in it, is used for cooking and as a dressing on both raw and cooked caribou. Berries are also beaten into properly aged caribou meat and the whole frozen until it is consumed, generally raw. This is also called kwak.

Discussion

The area in which this study was conducted is basically a north-sloping tundra. Annual rainfall is 4–8″. Temperature maximums are 46 to 62°; minimums are 16 to 22°. The area is underlain by permafrost (Arnold *et al.*, 1968). We did not expect to find much plant utilization by native peoples there. Those recent reports available to us supported this conclusion (Ford, 1959; Spencer and Jennings, 1965; Arnold *et al.*, 1968). Murdoch (1892) remarked that "few plants of any service to man grow in this region." His company could find no fruit that could be eaten and noted only the cranberry (*Vaccinium vitis-idaea*) growing near Barrow. Even it produced no fruit during either season in which they were in residence (1882-1883). He recorded that a bright pink *Pedicularis* was one of the few plants specifically named by the Eskimos and that it was called "maisun." This name seems close to "masu" (Table I), a term applied to several roots, including species of the genus *Pedicularis.* Murdoch further stated: "We saw this people eat no vegetable substances, though they informed us that the buds of the willow were sometimes eaten." This dish is presently referred to as "okpik" (Tables II-V) and has, according to our findings, rather wide usage.

Another reference to the lack of vegetation in the Eskimo diet concerned reindeer stomach (rumen) contents, which are mostly fermented lichens. The excised rumen is allowed to "ripen" for 2 or 3 days before its contents are consumed. Murdoch stated that his expedition "saw and heard nothing of this habit, so generally noted among Eskimos and in Siberia" but did note "their preference for fresh feces of deer." The animal he referred to is probably caribou, a wild American reindeer which today exists in Alaska in phenomenally large herds. We noted no such affinity for fecal matter by present Eskimos. Each Eskimo family with dogs, according to our informant Mr. Pete Sovalik, takes about 75 caribou each year. It is, therefore, possible to regard such an item as caribou rumen contents, consisting mostly of lichens and bacteria, as a fairly regular dietary constituent. Such a dietary item, even in small quantities, could well supply a high percentage of many vitamins because of bacterial syntheses during fermentation. We have not, however, performed any analyses to determine the vitamin levels in this material.

The use of clay as a dietary item was intriguing to us. The clay employed came primarily from a single inland location, Umiat, a now deserted site, and families who used it made the trip every few years to replenish their supply. It is a montmorillonite called Umiat Bentonite (Anderson and Reynolds, 1966), and was spoken of by many of our informants as being "sweet" to the taste. Bentonite clays also have a high ability to absorb toxic substances (Smith *et al.,* 1967). Minnich *et al.* (1968) reported that the use of such items in the diet was detrimental to iron absorption in humans. One effect of iron deficiency, Plummer-Vinson syndrome, may be minimized by increased absorption of iron from the gastro-intestinal tract resulting from high ascorbic acid (Vitamin C) intake. This vitamin could be obtained from fresh or quick-frozen plants.

Man *et al.* (1962), in their study of the health and nutritional status of some Alaskan Eskimos, concluded that specific nutritional deficiencies were not a health problem at that time (1958). This study also pointed out two dietary "riddles" of the Eskimo. One was that intake of Vitamin C was low, but scurvy was not seen. These investigators attributed this fact to "sporadic intake of a few exceptionally rich sources of vitamin C—for example, willow leaves and cloudberries—aided by effective if unpremeditated ways of preserving these during the winter." The other concerned clinical manifestations of Vitamin A deficiency, even though many items in the diet contained high levels of vitamin A. Lack of voucher specimens and scientific identifications of their plants make comparisons with our plant collections tenuous.

Berries and seal oil were, until quite recently, major items of reciprocal trade between inland and coastal Eskimos (Spencer, 1959; Arnold *et al.*, 1968). Hence in inland North Alaska, seal oil was a common preservative of all plant parts, and inland plant products were a common part of the diets of coastal Eskimos. Seal oil is itself a good source of Vitamin A, but only when fresh. These plant-oil mixtures are high in Vitamin C, but lose Vitamin A rapidly upon aging (Mann *et al.*, 1962).

An implication of these dietary riddles is that the casual use of plants is far more important in the Eskimo diet than their quantity or regularity of use would indicate. Several food plants were definitely present at each of the village sites we visited, in spite of the fact that these same plants were seldom mentioned as food sources by other authors or by the Eskimos themselves (Murdoch, 1892; Spencer, 1959; Spencer and Jennings, 1965). A similar situation exists among the Chocó, a primitive riverbank-dwelling tribe in Panama's Province of Darièn. There the major food crops are upland rice (*Oryza sativa*) and platano (*Musa paradisiaca*), but the dooryards contain upward of 50 other useful plants. These cultivars furnish leaves, roots, or fruits which are consumed in only small amounts and at sporadic intervals, yet they apparently serve as sources of vitamins in an otherwise restricted diet (Covich and Nickerson, 1966).

The Eskimo culture is in the process of change. The

continued opportunity for steady employment at *DEW-line* sites and at research sites, such as the Arctic Research Laboratory east of Barrow, has meant a shift in the population patterns of the Eskimo from many small villages to a few larger ones, especially Barrow, with the consequence of incipient environmental pollution. Centrally managed schools at Barrow, Wainwright, Koktuvik, and Anaktuvuk Pass, coupled with a growing awareness among the older Eskimos of the handicap imposed by a lack of education in coping with the modern changes that have been introduced into the Arctic, have speeded up this change. Nowhere is change more marked than in dietary habits, which in some cases have been completely altered from Eskimo (native) foods to "tunnik" (white man) foods. Of course these latter foods must be brought into the villages from outside. Relatively high wages with little in the way of native goods to purchase have abetted this dependence on the outside for food. Therefore, a shift has occurred from high-protein to a high-carbohydrate diet. The possibilities of long-term research concerning the effects wrought on human beings by such a change have apparently not yet been seriously explored, even though they were pointed out in 1962 by Mann *et al.*

The forces of acculturation are deleting the several ways in which the Eskimo utilized the limited plant resources of his environment as positive survival factors from his life and skills. The existing correlations between age and the knowledge of native plants, as shown in Figure 3, bear out this contention. At the same time, such forces provide us with a singular opportunity to observe their effects on these human populations in so-called simple ecosystems, as well as the effects upon the ecosystems themselves. Comparative studies have been done by Hansen (1966, 1967) and Hansen *et al.* (1966), which dealt with radioactivity

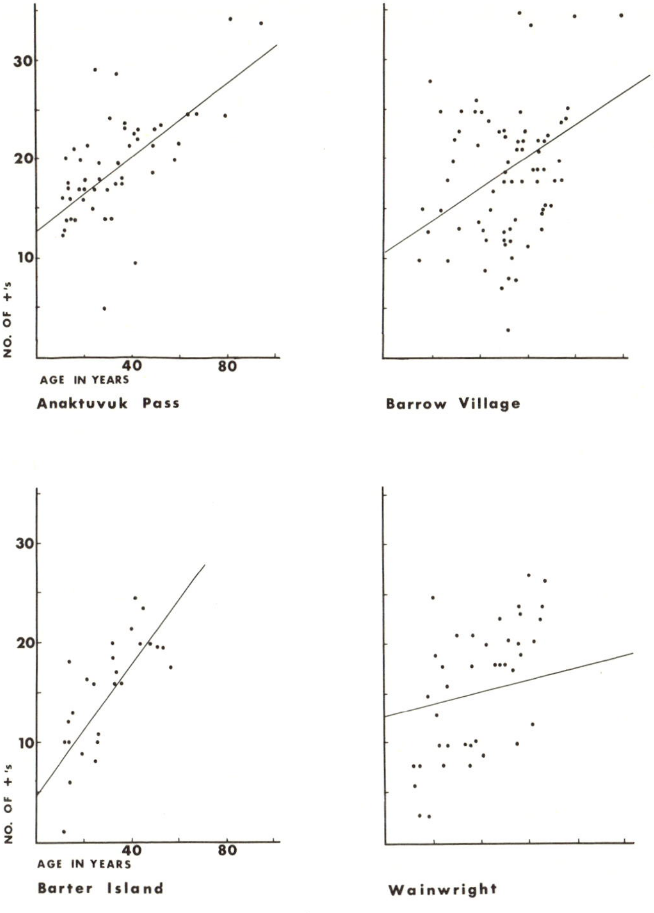

Fig. 3

Linear regressions of amount of knowledge about native flora on age of individuals. A positive slope indicates that old individuals know more about their native flora than young individuals.

The equations for these respective lines are given below:

ANAKTUVUK PASS	$y = .186x + 12.87$
BARROW VILLAGE	$y = .156x + 10.98$
BARTER ISLAND	$y = .310x + 4.78$
WAINWRIGHT	$y = 0.59x + 12.66$

levels and Cesium-137 body burdens in native populations consistently utilizing native foods versus those consistently utilizing imported foods. Such studies, however, are rare.

With the recent (1969) discovery of oil under the Arctic Slope, these acculturating forces can only be speeded up. Studies designed to measure closely the impact of these forces on all Arctic ecosystems and the human beings inhabiting them must soon be started if there are to be any reliable base-lines with which the inevitable changes may be compared.

REFERENCES

Anderson, D. M., and Reynolds, R. C., 1966. "Umiat Bentonite: An Unusual Montmorillonite from Umiat, Alaska," *The American Mineralogist.* 51: 1443-1456.

Anderson, J. P., 1959. *A Flora of Alaska and Adjacent Parts of Canada.* Iowa State College, Ames. 375 pp.

Arnold, D., Hickock, D. M., and Wannicke, E. C., 1968. *Alaska Natives and the Land* (Anchorage U.S.G.P.O.) 565 pp.

Covich, A. P., and Nickerson, N. H., 1966. "Studies of Cultivated Plants in Chocó Dwelling Clearings, Darièn, Panama," *Econ. Bot.* 20: 285-301.

Ford, James A., 1959. *Eskimo Prehistory in the Vicinity of Point Barrow, Alaska.* Anthropology Paper No. 17. American Museum of Natural History. New York. 285 pp.

Hanson, Wayne C., 1966. "Radioecological concentration processes characterizing Arctic ecosystems," *Radioecological Concentration Processes.* Pergamon Press, New York: 183-191.

———, 1967. "Cesium-137 in Alaskan Lichens, Caribou, and Eskimos." *Health Physics* 13: 383-389.

———, Watson, D. G., and Perkins, R. W., 1966. "Concentration and retention of fallout radionuclides in Alaskan arctic ecosystems," *Radioecological Concentration Processes.* Pergamon Press, New York: 233-245.

Mann, G. V., Scott, E. M., Hursh, L. M., Heller, C. A., Youmans, J. B., Comsolazio, C. F., Bridgeforth, E. B., Russell, A. L., Silverman, M., and eleven technical assistants, 1962. "The Health and Nutritional Status of Alaskan Eskimos," *American Journal of Clinical Nutrition* 11: 31-76.

Minnich, V., Okcuoglu, A., Tarcon, Y., Arcasoy, A., Cin, S., Yorukoglu, O., Renda, F., and Demirag, B., 1968. "Pica in Turkey II—Effect of Clay upon Iron Absorption," *American Journal of Clinical Nutrition* 21: 78-86.

Murdoch, John, 1892. *Ethnological Results of the Point Barrow Expedition, 1881-1883.* Accompanying papers 1, 9th Annual Report, Bureau of (American) Ethnology. Washington, D.C. 441 pp.

Nickerson, N. H., and Covich, A. P., 1966. "A Collection of Maize from Darièn, Panama," *Econ. Bot.* 20: 434-440.

Rowe, N. H., and Johnson, C. N., 1964. "A Search for the Burkitt Lymphoma in tropical Central America." *British Journal of Cancer* 18: 228-232.

Rowe, N. H., Watson, F. R., Nickerson, N. H., and Richter, E. A., 1969. "Environmental Influences upon Salivary Gland Carcinogenesis," Paper given at the International Conf. on Dental Diseases, Johannesburg, South Africa. July, 1969.

Sexton, O. J., Heatwole, H., and Knight, D., 1964. "Correlation of Micro-Distribution of Some Panamanian Reptiles and Amphibians with Structural Organization of Habitat." *Caribbean Journal of Science* 4: 261-295.

Shishmaref Day School Students, Shishmaref, Alaska, 1952. *Eskimo Cookbook.* Alaska Crippled Children's Association, Anchorage, Alaska. 36 pp.

Smith, R. P., Gosselin, R. E., Henderson, J., and Anderson, D. N., 1967. "Comparison of the Adsorptive Properties of Activated Charcoal and Alaskan Montmorillonite for Some Common Poisons." *Toxicology and Applied Pharmacology* 10: 95-104.

Spencer, Robert F., 1959. *The North Alaskan Eskimo—A Study in Ecology and Society.* Smithsonian Institute Bureau of American Ethnology, Bulletin 171. 440 pp.

Spencer, Robert F., Jennings, Jesse D., *et al.*, 1965. *The Native Americans.* Harper & Row, New York. 539 pp.

Stamp, L. Dudley, 1965. *The Geography of Life and Death,* Cornell University Press. Ithaca, N.Y. 160 pp.

Stoney, George M., 1899. *Navy Explorations in Alaska.* U.S. Naval Institute Proceedings, Annapolis 25: 533-584 and 799-849.

Wiggins, J. L., and Thomas, J. H., 1962. *A Flora of the Alaskan Arctic Slope.* A.I.N.A. Publ. No. 4. University of Toronto Press. 425 pp.

E. O. Callen

DIETARY PATTERNS IN MEXICO BETWEEN 6500 B.C. AND 1580 A.D.

Archaeologists speak of ancient man in the New World as going through stages of cultural development. When he first crossed the Bering land bridge, he was in the hunting or paleo-Indian stage. This was followed in turn by a food-gathering stage, an incipient agriculture stage, and finally, a stage where the economy was based on full-time agriculture. Because of the rapid increase in knowledge, it has become more and more difficult to draw a sharp distinction between these stages. Consequently, we now speak of a primitive hunting stage, followed by a long stage of food-gathering and incipient agriculture, terminating with the appearance of pottery, which marks the beginning of full-time agriculture (MacNeish 1964).

In Mexico the change from the hunting stage to that of food-gathering and incipient agriculture occurred just before 7000 BC. (MacNeish l.c.). At about that time, there seems to have been a distinct warming trend in the climate, which resulted in some areas of Mexico becoming so dry that they developed either a mesquite or a thorn-scrub/cactus vegetation. Because of the dryness, the preservation of biological materials was excellent. Animal droppings and human feces (called coprolites) were rapidly desiccated when exposed to the air, and when recovered by the archaeologist, they look as if they had been freeze-dried by the most modern of methods. A number of years ago I devised a method of reconstituting these desiccated coprolites, so that undigested plant fragments could be identified microscopically (Callen and Cameron 1955; Callen 1960). To date I have been able to identify twenty-three plants to genus, and another five to family (Fig. 1).

In this paper I plan to confine myself to results from two sites in Mexico, the Ocampo Caves in Tamaulipas State and the Tehuacan Caves of Puebla State, some 400 miles apart.

In the Ocampo Caves of NE Mexico, in a dry mesquite area, the earliest coprolites were obtained from Level 7 of

PLANTS IDENTIFIED FROM COPROLITES FOUND IN PERU, TAMAULIPAS & TEHUACAN CAVES

AGAVE	PHASEOLUS
ALOE	PHYSALIS
AMARANTHUS	PROSOPIS
CANAVALIA	SETARIA
CARTHAMNUS	TILLANDSIA USNEOIDES
CEIBA	TILLANDSIA sp.
CUCURBITA	ZEA
DIOSPYROS	ZIZYPHUS
HELIANTHUS	YUCCA
LAGENARIA	other beans
LEMAIREOCEREUS	other cactus seeds
MANIHOT	other composite seeds
OPUNTIA	caryophyllaceous seeds
PANICUM	reeds

Fig. 1

the Infiernillo cultural phase of cave Tmc 248, dated at 6500 BC (Fig. 2), though the date shown in the figure is a median one for the two layers recorded there. This was close to the beginning of the food-gathering stage of paleo-Indian development. Fig. 2 shows the principal plants eaten together during several meals, a meal being defined as the plant and animal material churned up in the stomach together, and passed into and through the intestine together. *Opuntia* stems (rarely the fruits) and the leaves of *Agave,* parts of two readily propagated plants, plus the fruits of *Capsicum* and *Prosopis* constituted the principal plants of these meals. A root crop was absent from the list of plants eaten, and some form of animal protein (labeled "meat") was eaten in four of the six meals shown. Beans

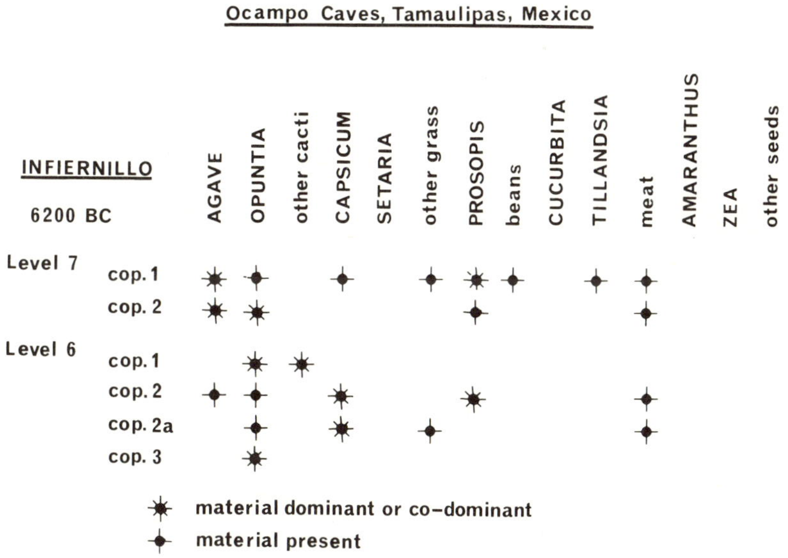

Fig. 2

were present in the diet, but it has not proved possible to identify the genus, because the characteristics by which this could be done are generally destroyed in the eating process. From the rubbish of the cave floor, MacNeish (1964) who excavated these caves, gives the Infiernillo diet as consisting of 50% from hunting and trapping meat, 49% from collecting wild plants, and 1% from cultivating plants.

The next cultural phase, Ocampo, has four levels spanning some 2300 years. MacNeish (l.c.) judged that hunting had decreased, that plant collecting had greatly increased, and that incipient agriculture had grown only slightly. The coprolites show that in Level 5 (Fig. 3), the oldest Ocampo level at roughly 4000 BC, the single most important plant

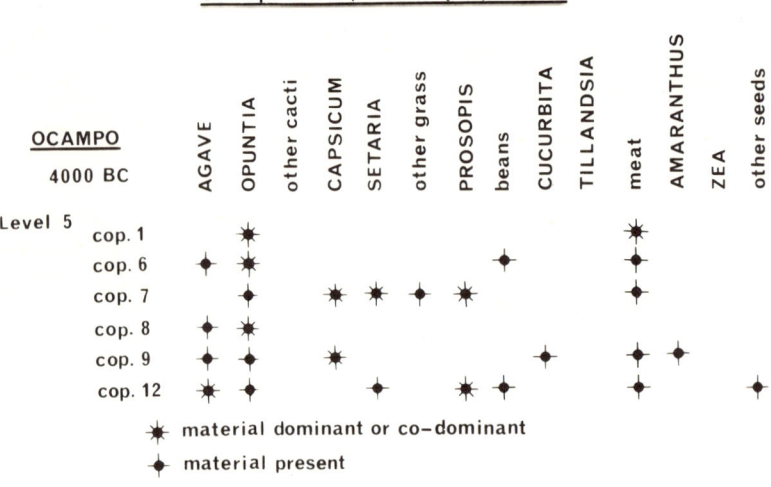

Ocampo Caves, Tamaulipas, Mexico

OCAMPO 4000 BC		AGAVE	OPUNTIA	other cacti	CAPSICUM	SETARIA	other grass	PROSOPIS	beans	CUCURBITA	TILLANDSIA	meat	AMARANTHUS	ZEA	other seeds
Level 5	cop. 1		✱									✱			
	cop. 6	✦	✱						✦			✦			
	cop. 7		✦		✱	✱	✦	✱				✦			
	cop. 8	✦	✱												
	cop. 9	✦	✦		✱					✦		✦	✦		
	cop. 12	✱	✦			✦		✱	✦			✦			✦

✱ material dominant or co-dominant

✦ material present

Fig. 3

Ocampo Caves, Tamaulipas, Mexico

OCAMPO

3800 BC

Level 4a	AGAVE	OPUNTIA	other cacti	CAPSICUM	SETARIA	other grass	PROSOPIS	beans	CUCURBITA	TILLANDSIA	meat	AMARANTHUS	ZEA	other seeds
cop. 2	✱	✱	◆					◆		✱	◆			◆
cop. 3	◆	✱		◆		✱					✱			
cop. 4	◆	◆		◆		✱		◆						
cop. 6	✱	◆		◆		◆		✱			✱			◆
cop. 7	◆						✱				✱			◆
cop 8	✱	✱				◆	◆	◆			◆			

✱ material dominant or co-dominant

◆ material present

Fig. 4

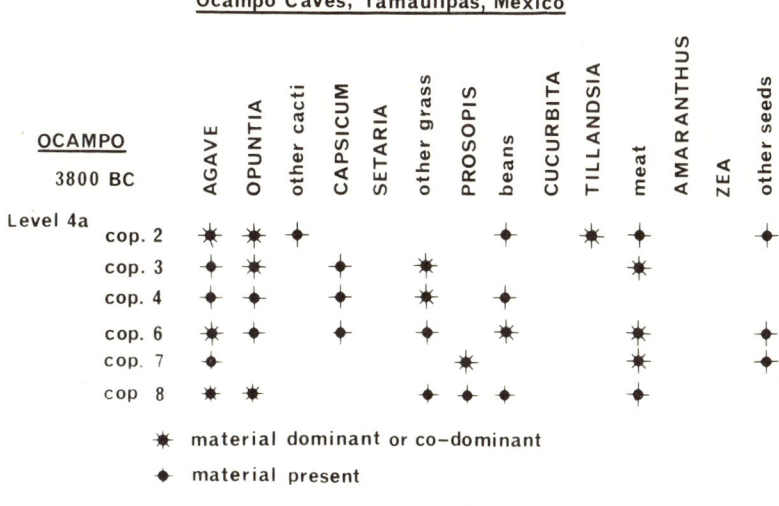

was *Opuntia,* with meat and then *Agave* as the next most frequently eaten items. At this level, *Setaria, Cucurbita,* and *Amaranthus* appear in the coprolites for the first time. In Level 4a (Fig. 4) at 3800 BC, *Agave* and *Opuntia* were again the main plants, with meat still a very important item. Level 4 (Fig. 5) at 3650 BC still has *Agave* and *Opuntia* as important items, though meat much less so. The youngest Ocampo level is Level 9 from a neighboring cave, Tmc 247, at about 2600 BC (not shown). Here *Agave* was the most important and frequently eaten plant, followed in order by *Prosopis, Setaria,* and then *Opuntia.*

According to MacNeish (l.c.) the next two cultural phases, Flacco and Guerra, show an increase in the amount of incipient agriculture at the expense of hunting and trapping, and of food-gathering. This was not sudden, he pointed out, but really a slow accumulation of more and more domesticated plants replacing the wild plant foodstuffs. Looking at the coprolites of the Flacco phase at approximately 1950 BC (Fig. 6), Level 3 of cave Tmc 248 again shows *Agave* as the principal plant of the diet, with *Capsicum* and *Setaria* as the next most frequently eaten ones, and meat an important item in some. However, that is only in the six representative coprolites shown. When the 58 coprolites analysed for Level 3 were summarized (Fig. 9), *Prosopis* was the second most frequently eaten item, followed by *Capsicum* and meat. For the Guerra cultural phase, Level 4b, of cave Tmc 247, at roughly 1600

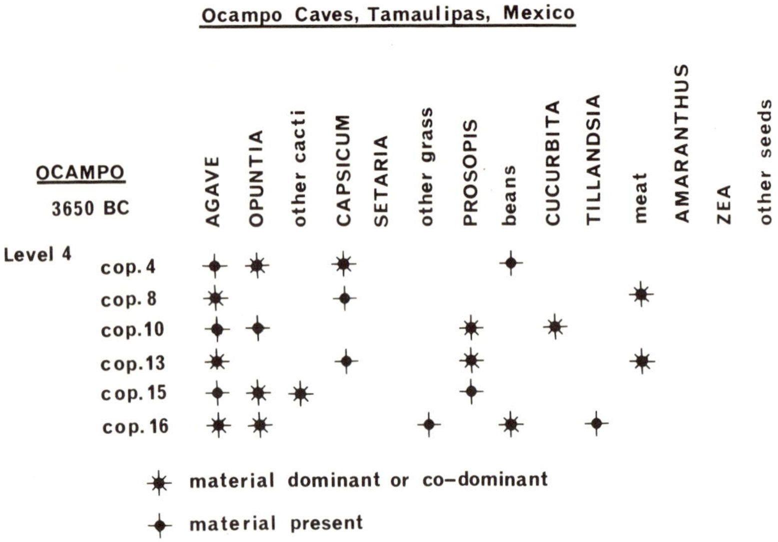

Fig. 5

Ocampo Caves, Tamaulipas, Mexico

FLACCO
1950 BC

Level 3		AGAVE	OPUNTIA	other cacti	CAPSICUM	SETARIA	other grass	PROSOPIS	beans	CUCURBITA	TILLANDSIA	meat	AMARANTHUS	ZEA	other seeds
	cop. 4	✱			✦	✦	✦	✦				✱			
	cop. 13	✦	✦	✦	✱	✦			✦						
	cop. 20	✦			✦	✱			✦			✱			
	cop. 22	✱			✦			✱				✱			
	cop. 44	✦			✱	✱									
	cop. 58	✱			✦	✦		✱	✦		✱				

✱ material dominant or co-dominant
✦ material present

Fig. 6

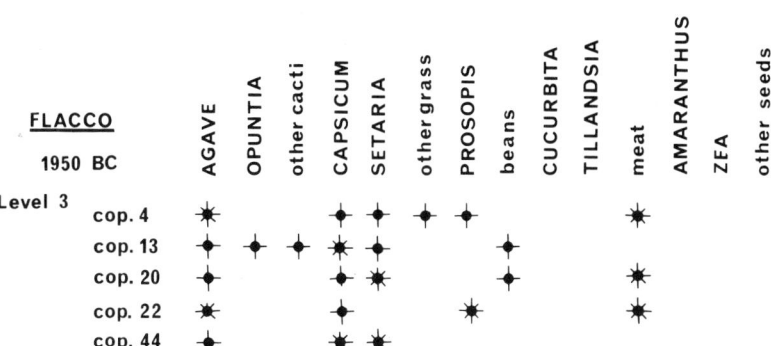

BC (Fig. 9), *Agave,* meat, and *Prosopis* were the three principal items of the meals.

The coprolites from the succeeding cultural phase, Mesa de Guaje, also came from cave Tmc 247, and here the picture is not quite so clear (Fig. 7). According to MacNeish (1964), the transition from incipient to full-time village agriculture in the Tamaulipas caves was somewhat behind areas farther south in Middle America. This means, therefore, that in Mesa de Guaje, Levels 4 and 4a (Figs. 9 and 7 respectively) must still be considered as belonging to the end of the incipient agriculture stage of development. In Levels 4 and 4a, *Agave* was the principal plant eaten, followed by *Prosopis.* Some form of meat protein was eaten at practically all meals. Meanwhile, *Opuntia* had

Ocampo Caves, Tamaulipas, Mexico

MESA DE GUAJE 1200 BC		AGAVE	OPUNTIA	other cacti	CAPSICUM	SETARIA	other grass	PROSOPIS	beans	CUCURBITA	TILLANDSIA	meat	AMARANTHUS	ZEA	other seed
Level 4a	cop. 6							✱				✦			
	cop. 22	✦	✱	✱	✦	✦		✦	✦	✦	✦	✱			✦
	cop. 36					✱						✱		✱	
	cop. 43	✱			✦			✱	✦			✱			
	cop. 52	✱				✱						✦	✦		✦
	cop. 57	✦		✱				✦	✦	✱		✱			

✱ material dominant or co-dominant

✦ material present

Fig. 7

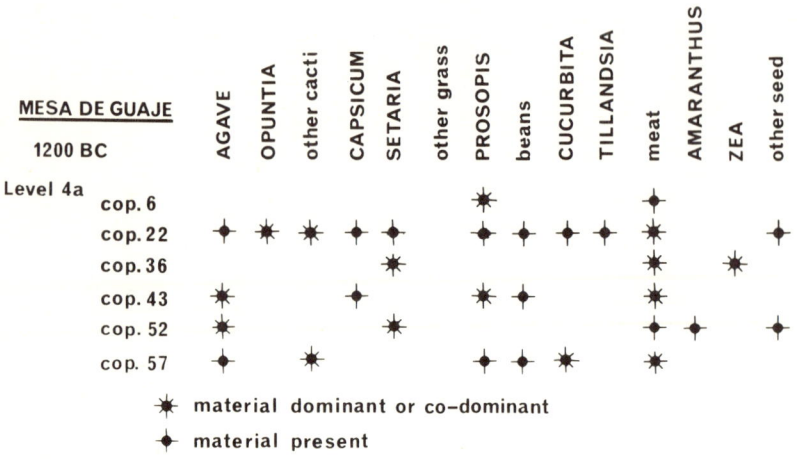

become much less important than it had been in the diet 5000 years before.

There is a considerable gap until the San Lorenzo cultural phase at roughly 1450 AD (Fig. 8), as no coprolites were recovered from the intervening period. According to MacNeish (1958), in this phase there had been a definite decay in the culture of these peoples; however, as we can see from Fig. 8, in their diet they were still eating the same plants as their ancestors, but with different emphases. Instead of cacti of several kinds and *Agave,* there was a great reliance on meat protein, seeds, and fruits. Cacti (incl. *Opuntia*) were probably only eaten to make up bulk.

The results from the two Ocampo Caves are summarized in Fig. 9. In 6500 BC *Opuntia* was the most frequently

Ocampo Caves, Tamaulipas, Mexico

SAN LORENZO 1450 AD		AGAVE	OPUNTIA	other cacti	CAPSICUM	SETARIA	other grass	PROSOPIS	beans	CUCURBITA	TILLANDSIA	meat	AMARANTHUS	ZEA	other seeds
Level 2	cop. 2		✦			✦		✦		✱		✱			✱
	cop. 3	✦	✦		✦	✦	✦	✦		✦		✱			✱
	cop. 9	✦	✱	✦		✦	✦	✱			✦	✱		✦	✦
	cop. 17			✦	✱	✱		✦				✱			
	cop. 22		✱		✱	✦									
	cop. 27	✦		✦	✦		✦	✱				✱		✦	✦

✱ material dominant or co-dominant

✦ material present

Fig. 8

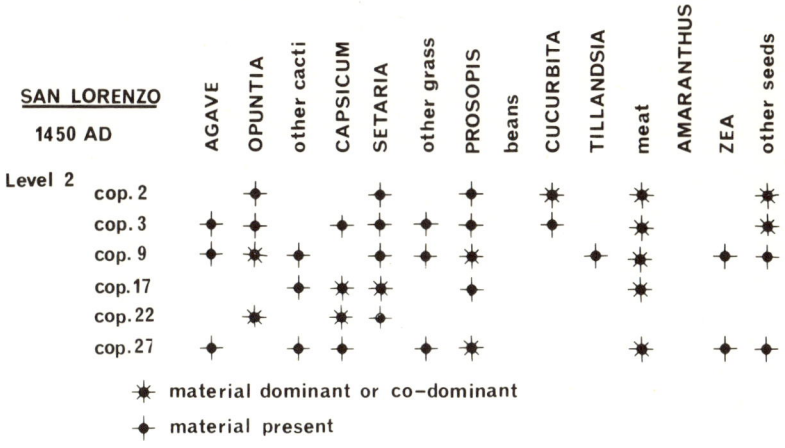

eaten plant, and remained so for over 3000 years, but after 3600 BC it gradually lost importance. *Agave,* which was the second most important plant in 6500 BC, took over as the most important one in 3600 BC, only in turn to lose favor and be replaced by meat and, subsequently, other plants, as the time of the Spanish Conquest approached.

In the Tehuacan Caves in South Central Mexico, an area of thorn-scrub/cactus vegetation, the earliest coprolites were obtained from a layer of the El Riego cultural phase in cave Tc 50, dated at approximately 6500 BC (Fig. 10). These are believed to be from early in the food-gathering stage. Here the chief plants eaten were *Setaria* (a grass) and the starchy roots of the *Ceiba* tree. Cacti other than *Opuntia* and *Lemaireocereus,* other grasses, and meat were

Ocampo Caves, Tamaulipas, Mexico

Plants eaten : in order of frequency

Infiernillo		
248 Level 7/6	6200 BC	OPUNTIA, meat, AGAVE – CAPSICUM – PROSOPIS, beans
Ocampo		
248 Level 5	4000 BC	OPUNTIA, meat, CAPSICUM, AGAVE, beans
248 Level 4a	3800 BC	OPUNTIA – AGAVE, meat, CAPSICUM – beans
248 Level 4	3650 BC	AGAVE, OPUNTIA, CAPSICUM, PROSOPIS – beans, meat
247 Level 9	2600 BC	AGAVE – PROSOPIS, OPUNTIA – CAPSICUM – beans – meat
Flacco		
248 Level 3	1950 BC	AGAVE – PROSOPIS, CAPSICUM, meat, OPUNTIA
Guerra		
247 Level 4b	1600 BC	AGAVE – meat, PROSOPIS, beans, SETARIA

Mesa de Guaje		
247 Level 4	1400 BC	AGAVE, PROSOPIS, OPUNTIA – SETARIA, beans – CUCURBITA, meat
247 Level 4a	1200 BC	meat, AGAVE, PROSOPIS, beans, OPUNTIA, TILLANDSIA, CAPSICUM
San Lorenzo		
247 Level 2	1450 AD	PROSOPIS, meat, cacti, AGAVE, CAPSICUM – seeds, OPUNTIA

Carbon–14 dating

Fig. 9

Tehuacan Caves, Puebla, Mexico

EL RIEGO Tc 50 5700 BC	CEIBA	SETARIA	AGAVE	OPUNTIA	LEMAIREOCEREUS	other cacti	PROSOPIS	DIOSPYROS	CAPSICUM	other grass	other seeds	meat	ZEA	beans
Zone XVI cop. 1		✱					✦		✦	✦		✦	✦	
XV cop. 2	✦	✱				✦				✦		✦	✦	
XIV cop. 4	✱	✱				✦				✦	✦	✦		
cop. 5	✱	✱				✦	✦			✦		✦		
cop. 6	✱	✱	✦		✦	✦			✦	✦				
cop. 7	✱		✦									✦	✦	

✱ material dominant or co-dominant

✦ material present

Fig. 10

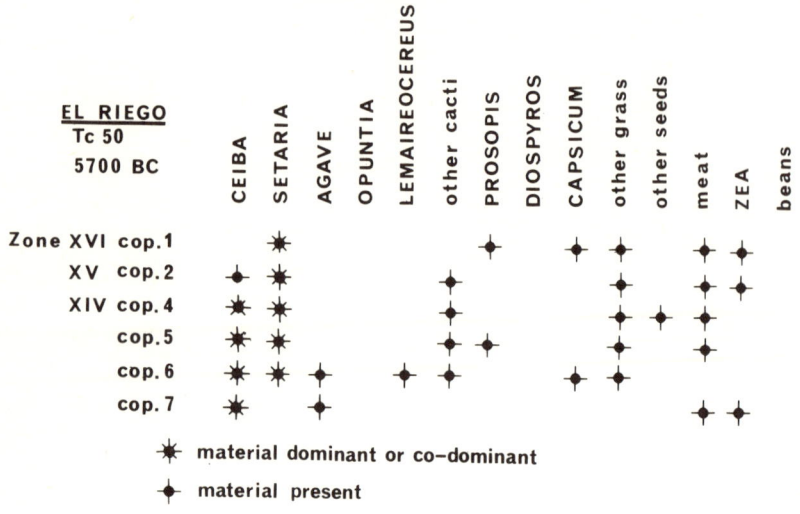

also eaten regularly. The records for *Zea* are still somewhat questionable. These are not seeds, but what I believe are fragments of leaf or husk of what was then still a wild plant (Mangelsdorf 1964). According to MacNeish (1967), the diet consisted of 41% wild plants, 5% cultivated ones, and 54% meat, as determined from all sources other than the coprolites.

In the next culture, the Coxcatlan phase, at approximately 4200 BC (Fig. 11), *Setaria* and *Ceiba* were still the principal plants of the diet, with some meat at practically every meal. According to MacNeish, the Coxcatlan diet consisted of 41% wild plants, 5% cultivated ones, and 54% meat, as determined from all sources other than the coprolites.

Relatively few coprolites were recovered from several succeeding phases covering a period of 2500 years, as the main cave (Tc 50) was uninhabited for much of that time. However, from neighboring caves we can see (Fig. 16) that meat and *Agave* leaves, grass seeds, *Prosopis* pods, and *Lemaireocereus* and *Opuntia* stems were all important in the diet. For the Abejas phase, MacNeish assesses the diet as consisting of 49% wild plants, 21% cultivated plants, and 30% meat; and the Ajalpan diet as 18% wild plants, 55% cultivated plants, and 27% meat. This latter was definitely an agricultural economy.

By the Santa Maria phase (550 BC), the main cave, Tc 50, was reoccupied (Fig. 12), and shows that the *Setaria*/*Ceiba* diet was as popular as ever, although this was a time of full agriculture. According to MacNeish, the Santa Maria

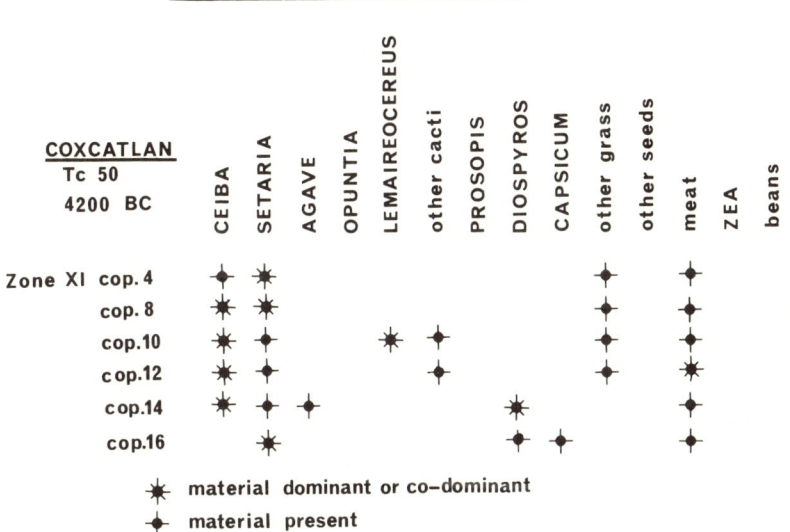

Tehuacan Caves, Puebla, Mexico

COXCATLAN Tc 50 4200 BC	CEIBA	SETARIA	AGAVE	OPUNTIA	LEMAIREOCEREUS	other cacti	PROSOPIS	DIOSPYROS	CAPSICUM	other grass	other seeds	meat	ZEA	beans
Zone XI cop. 4	✦	✱								✦		✦		
cop. 8	✱	✱								✦		✦		
cop.10	✱	✦			✱	✦				✦		✦		
cop.12	✱	✦				✦				✦		✱		
cop.14	✱	✦	✦					✱				✦		
cop.16		✱						✦	✦			✦		

✱ material dominant or co–dominant
✦ material present

Fig. 11

Tehuacan Caves, Puebla, Mexico

SANTA MARIA
Tc 50
550 BC

	CEIBA	SETARIA	AGAVE	OPUNTIA	LEMAIREOCEREUS	other cacti	PROSOPIS	DIOSPYROS	CAPSICUM	other grass	other seeds	meat	ZEA	beans
Zone VII cop. 4	✱	✱					✦	✦		✦				
cop. 8	✱	✦				✱	✦			✦	✦	✦	✦	
cop. 10	✱	✦			✦	✦	✦					✦		
cop.17		✱	✦				✦		✦	✦		✦		✦
cop.19		✦	✱				✦	✱				✦		
cop. 21	✦	✦			✱		✦					✦		

✱ material dominant or co-dominant
✦ material present

Fig. 12

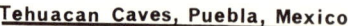

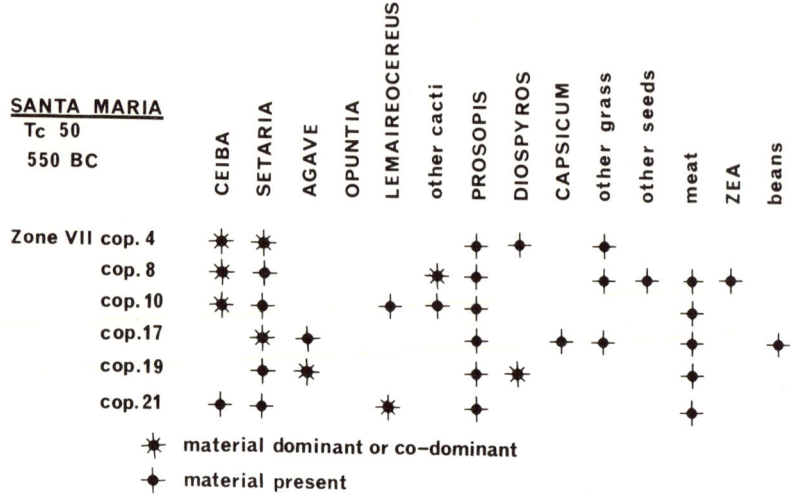

diet consisted of 17% wild plants, 58% cultivated plants, and 25% meat.

During the classic period (Palo Blanco phase) and the Christian era (Fig. 13), the *Setaria/Ceiba* diet was just as popular with the inhabitants of Tc 50 as it had been 7000 years before, though with other plants added, and with some meat at just about every meal. In two neighboring caves (Fig. 14), *Agave* and various cacti were the principal plants eaten, more or less as is seen in the earlier Abejas and Ajalpan phases. MacNeish assessed the Palo Blanco diet as consisting of 17% wild plants, 65% cultivated plants, and 18% meat.

During the post classic Venta Salada (Fig. 15), at roughly 1120 AD, there is considerable evidence of a decline in culture. *Agave,* cacti, beans, *Setaria,* and other grasses were

Tehuacan Caves, Puebla, Mexico

PALO BLANCO
Tc 50
250 AD

	CEIBA	SETARIA	AGAVE	OPUNTIA	LEMAIREOCEREUS	other cacti	PROSOPIS	DIOSPYROS	CAPSICUM	other grass	other seeds	meat	ZEA	beans
Zone VI cop. 19	✱		✦						✦	✦	✦	✦		
VI cop. 23	✱	✦	✦				✦	✱	✦	✦		✦		✦
VI cop. 26	✦	✦			✦	✱		✱		✦		✦		
VI cop. 30	✱	✦	✱	✦	✦	✦	✦			✦	✦	✦		✦
Zone IV cop. 95	✱	✦		✦	✦	✱				✦		✦		✦
IV cop. 98	✱	✦		✱								✦		✦

✱ material dominant or co-dominant

✦ material present

Fig. 13

Tehuacan Caves, Puebla, Mexico

PALO BLANCO
250 AD

	CEIBA	SETARIA	AGAVE	OPUNTIA	LEMAIREOCEREUS	other cacti	PROSOPIS	DIOSPYROS	CAPSICUM	other grass	other seeds	meat	ZEA	beans
Tc 254														
cop. 6			✱		✦	✦	✦					✦		
cop. 12			✱			✦						✦		
cop. 87				✦		✱	✱			✦	✦			
Tc 272														
cop. 55			✦	✦	✦	✱			✦	✦		✱	✦	✦
cop. 58			✦						✱		✦	✱		✦
cop. 67			✱	✱					✦			✦		

✱ material dominant or co-dominant

✦ material present

Fig. 14

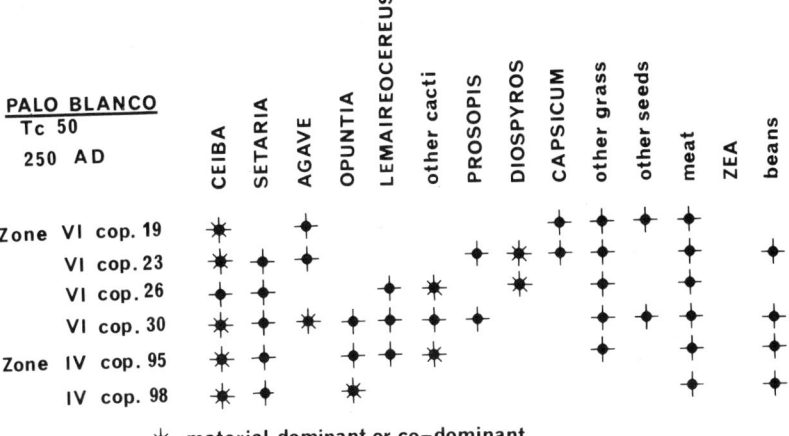

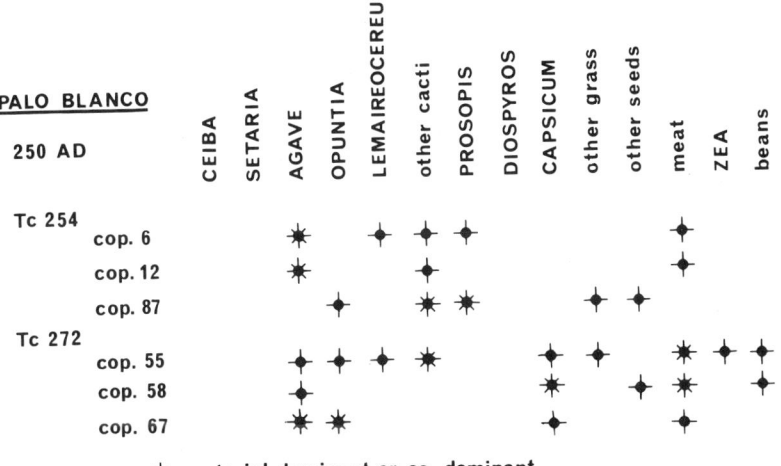

Tehuacan Caves, Puebla, Mexico

VENTA SALADA Tc 50 1120 AD		CEIBA	SETARIA	AGAVE	OPUNTIA	LEMAIREOCEREUS	other cacti	PROSOPIS	DIOSPYROS	CAPSICUM	other grass	other seed	meat	ZEA	beans
Zone III	cop. 26					✱	✦						✱		
	cop. 46			✱									✦		✱
	cop. 84	✦	✱												
Zone II	cop. 22			✱			✦						✦		✱
	cop. 80					✱									
Zone I	cop. 77	✦	✦	✱											

✱ material dominant or co–dominant

✦ material present

Fig. 15

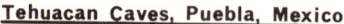

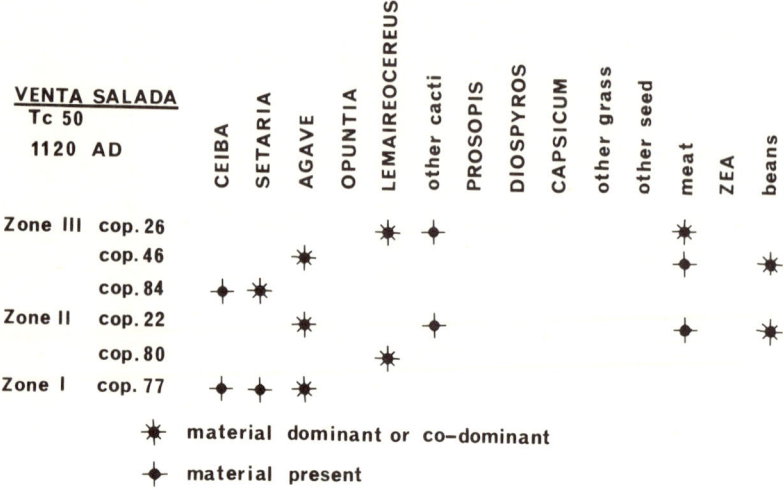

the principal plants of the diet. MacNeish summarized the diet as consisting of 8% wild plants, 75% cultivated plants, and 17% meat.

Summarizing the Tehuacan Cave diet as seen in the coprolites (Fig. 16), the main plants eaten over some 7000 years were *Ceiba, Setaria,* and other grasses, with *Agave* and meat becoming increasingly important. Various cacti, including *Opuntia* and *Lamaireocereus,* were always important items of the diet during this time.

It is evident that these cave diets (as distinct from town and city diets) were made up entirely of local plants, some of which must have been taken into cultivation. Comparing the most frequently eaten plants from both sets of caves, there are only three which do not occur in both (Fig. 17). These more southerly plants do not grow in Tamaulipas at present and probably did not in the past.

Tehuacan Caves, Puebla, Mexico

Plants eaten : in order of frequency

El Riego
5700 BC CEIBA – SETARIA – grass – cacti – meat, PROSOPIS – ZEA, AGAVE

Coxcatlan
4200 BC meat, CEIBA, SETARIA, grass, AGAVE, cacti – DIOSPYROS OPUNTIA

Abejas
2900 BC meat – grass, AGAVE – PROSOPIS – cacti, CEIBA – OPUNTIA – ZEA – DIOSPYROS, SETARIA

Ajalpan
1200 BC meat – AGAVE – LEMAIREOCEREUS, grass – cacti – beans – DIOSPYROS – seeds

Santa Maria
550 BC SETARIA, CEIBA – meat – PROSOPIS, grass, cacti – LEMAIREOCEREUS – DIOSPYROS

Palo Blanco
250 AD meat, AGAVE, grass, cacti, SETARIA, CEIBA, LEMAIREOCEREUS, PROSOPIS – beans

Venta Salada
1120 AD AGAVE, meat – cacti, beans, SETARIA – grass – LEMAIREOCEREUS, CEIBA – OPUNTIA

Fig. 16

PRINCIPAL PLANTS FROM TEHUACAN COPROLITES

PLANT	COMMON NAME	EATEN IN TAMAULIPAS
SETARIA	foxtail millet	yes
CEIBA	pochote	no
AGAVE	maguey	yes
OPUNTIA	prickly pear	yes
LEMAIREOCEREUS	organ cactus	no
other cacti	tuna	yes
DIOSPYROS	sapote	no
CUCURBITA	squash	yes
PROSOPIS	mesquite	yes
CAPSICUM	chili	yes
ZEA	maize	yes

Fig. 17

The surprising absence of maize and the relative unimportance of beans and squash are interesting. We know from the tribute lists that great quantities of these found their way to the main towns and the capital city. Perhaps the answer to their relative absence from the cave diet may be that these caves were used seasonally by the peasants and serfs, to sow, to tend, and to harvest the crops for town or tribute use. Some dog and ringtailed cat or coyote coprolites from the Santa Maria phase of the Tehuacan Cave Tc 50 contained fragments of cobs and almost complete maize grains, which suggests that the humans using the cave ate the plants growing near the cave, in the same way as their ancestors had done, and harvested the crop without eating any of it on the spot.

When I had nearly completed my analysis, Chadwick (1963) drew my attention to a Codex which recorded the plants eaten in many parts of Mexico between 1579 and 1581. King Philip II of Spain appointed a Commission in 1577, which framed a set of 50 questions to be answered by the elders and any Spaniards living in each principal town or city. Question XV involved the clothes they used to wear and now wear (1579-81), and which foods they ate in heathen times and which now. Some of these manuscripts were found in Madrid at the beginning of this century and were published by Francisco del Paso y Truncoso (1906).

The report for Tehuacan is missing, but those from the State of Oaxaca are found in vol. IV. Some of these towns (Teotitlan del Camino) are not more than 20 miles from the Tehuacan caves, and I have summarized the information in Fig. 18. To such information I have added material from a few other reports for localities near Mexico City published by Zelia Nuttall (1909). Knowing from the coprolites that the ancient diet included much *Agave* and *Opuntia,* I have placed them first in the list of foods, followed by herbs and roots. Evidently, the elders of some towns had knowledge going back only one or two generations. They said that they had always eaten what they ate now (1580). Perhaps, of course, they chose not to recall what their ancestors had eaten before the Conquest, or perhaps they had been town dwellers for many generations. But there were others who possessed knowledge stretching back hundreds and even thousands of years. They knew that "in ancient times their food consisted of cactus and cooked agave leaves, and some herbs of little nourishment, with which they lived healthily." Here then is documentary confirmation for the diet shown by my analysis of the coprolites. But I must emphasize again that

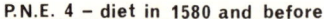

P.N.E. 4 – diet in 1580 and before

	cactus	agave	herbs	roots	tortillas, tamales	bread, maize bread	maize	beans	squash	chili	fruits	sage	amaranth	sweet potato	vegetables	wheat, barley	meat
Alcoman	●	●	●			✶	✶									✶	✶
Chinantla					✶	✶	●	✧	✶	✧	✶			✧			✧
Cuicatlan					●		✧	✧	✶		✶	●		✧			✧
Iztepexi					✧					✧							✶
Macuilsuchil		✶	●	●	✶		✧	✶	✶		✶	✶				✶	✶
Nochiztlan	✧						✧	✧	✶	✶	✶				✶	✶	✶
Tamazola	●		●		●		✧	✧	✧	✧	✶						✶
Tejupa					●							●					●
S. Juan Teotihuacan	✧	✧		●			✶	✶			✶		✶		✶	✶	✧
Teotitlan d. Camino							✧	✶	✶		✶		✶				✶
Teotitlan d. Valle			✧	●			✶	✶	✶		✧		✶			✶	✶
Tepechpan	●	●	●				✶	✶	✶	✶	✶	✶	✶		✶	✶	✶
Tepeucila					✧		✶	✧	✶	✧	✶				✶	✶	✧
Tequizistlan	✧	✧	●		✶	✶	✶	✶	✶	✶	✶	✶	✶			✶	✶
Teticpac			●	●			✶	✶	✶		✶	✶				✶	✶
Titlantongo	✧		●				✧	✧	✧	✧	✶				✶	✶	✧
Ucila							✧	✧		✧	✧				✶	✶	✶

● - pre 1580 ✶ - 1580 ✧ - 1580 and before

Fig. 18

this is a cave diet, originated in the earliest days of food-gathering and incipient agriculture, and retained by the peasants and slaves when they temporarily reinhabited the caves, even up to the time of the Spanish Conquest.

I have not referred to seasonality—that is dealt with in another place (Callen 1967, 1969)—nor have I attempted to define what constitutes a cultivated plant. I have only dealt with plants which were definitely eaten, as shown by coprolite analysis.

REFERENCES

Callen, E. O. 1960. "A Prehistoric Diet Revealed in Coprolites." *The New Scientist* 8 (190): 35-40.

———, 1967. "The First New World Cereal." *American Antiquity* 32 (4): 535-538.

———, 1968. "Analysis of the Tehuacan Coprolites." *The Prehistory of the Tehuacan Valley*, edit. Douglas S. Byers, Univ. of Texas Press, Austin, vol. 1, ch. 14: 261-289.

———, 1969. "Diet as revealed by coprolites." *Science in Archaeology*, edit. Don Brothwell and Eric Higgs, 2nd edition, Thames and Hudson, London.

Callen, E. O., and Cameron, T. W. M. 1955. "The Diet and Parasites of Prehistoric Huaca Prieta Indians as Determined by Dried Coprolites." *Proceedings of the Royal Society of Canada* 1955: 51 (abstr.).

Chadwick, R. L. 1963. "The God Malteutl in the Histoyre du Mechique." *Tlalocan* 4 (3): 264-270.

MacNeish, R. S. 1958. "Preliminary Archaeological Investigation in the Sierra de Tamaulipas, Mexico." *Transactions of the American Philosophical Society*, N.S. 48 (6): 1-210.

———, 1964. "Origins of agriculture in Middle America." *Handbook of Middle American Indians*, vol. 1, edit. Robert C. West, Univ. of Texas Press, Austin, ch. 13: 427-445.

MacNeish, R. S. 1968. "A Summary of the Subsistence." *The Prehistory of the Tehuacan Valley*, edit. Douglas S. Byers, Univ. of Texas Press, Austin, vol. 1, ch. 15: 290-309.

Mangelsdorf, P. C., MacNeish, R. S., and Walton, W. C. 1964. "Domestication of Corn." *Science* 143 (3606): 538-545.

Nuttall, Zelia. 1926. "Official Reports on the Towns of Tequizistlan, Tepechpan, Alcoman and San Juan Teotihuacan." *Papers of the Peabody Museum of Archaeology and Ethnology*, Harvard Univ. 11 (2): 39-84.

Paso y Truncoso, F. del. 1905. *Papales de Nueva Espana*, Sucs. de Rivandeneyra, Madrid, vol. 4: 1-231.

A. W. Williams

DIETARY PATTERNS IN THREE MEXICAN VILLAGES*

Although several important position papers have been published in recent years,[1] actual diets of contemporary people are not common in anthropological literature, nor are caloric-energy expenditure data on the production and consumption of food in human societies at all frequent.[2] The present study is a small contribution toward filling this gap, and its greatest merit may lie in the discussions that it may prompt. This study is presented with a plea for

* Research was supported by a National Science Foundation grant to Richard B. Woodbury; and by National Science Foundation grant GS 1616 to A.W. Williams and Kent Flannery (Co-principal Investigators).

1. See O. D. Duncan, "From Social System to Ecosystem," *Sociological Inquiry*, Vol. 31, p. 140–49, 1961; Clifford Geertz, *Agricultural Involution* (Berkeley: University of California Press, 1963); and Andrew P. Vayda, "Anthropologist and Ecological Problems," *Man, Culture, and Animals*, Anthony Leeds and Andrew P. Vayda, eds. (Washington, D.C.: American Association for the Advancement of Science, Pub. 78, 1965).

2. Notable exceptions include Roy Rappaport's superb analysis of the Tsembaba Maring, who are slash-and-burn farmers occupying a small territory in the Central Highlands of New Guinea (*Pigs for the Ancestors*, Yale University Press, 1968). Also, Moisés Behar's article,

help in designing better methods for gathering data on the individual diets of people in various cultures.

The data presented here were collected in three *mestizo* villages in south-central Mexico during three field seasons which spanned a 4-year period (1964-68). The impetus for getting information on dietary practices came from two sources: 1) a general interest in the theoretical proposition that as there is an increase in per capita energy in a human society, the society becomes more complex; and 2) the need to provide ethnographic data from villages utilizing irrigation in their farming activities for archeological analogs. Therefore, the central focus of the research was not diets exclusively, yet 130 daily diets of individuals were collected and the work patterns of individuals in the three villages were documented. In general it was learned that there was a high intake of corn products and vegetable protein and a low intake of animal protein, with an average daily caloric intake of 1,450 calories for the 130 individuals.

Most of the information concerning daily food intake was gathered during the months of June, July, and August; therefore, there is a summer bias. The summer eating pattern is offset somewhat by the fact that all three villages, Coxcatlan and Calipam in the State of Puebla, and San Gabriel Etla in the State of Oaxaca, seldom if ever have temperatures below freezing. Therefore, crops are grown in all 12 months of the year in each location; however, commercial crops such as sugar cane and alfalfa dominate the annual growing regime and use of the land. Sugar cane grows continuously and is cut once every 12

"Food and Nutrition of the Maya before the Conquest and the Present Time," in *Biomedical Challenges Presented by the American Indian* (Washington, D.C.: Pan American Health Organization, World Health Organization, Scientific Publication No. 165, 1968).

months in Coxcatlan and Calipam. Farmers in San Gabriel grow alfalfa throughout the entire year and are able to cut it every 40 days. The summer period is the main growing season; and fruits and vegetables such as apples, pears, papaya, mangoes, squash, corn, tomatoes, and chili are much more available during June, July, and August than in any other months of the year.

The three communities are rural villages in which farming is the dominant occupation of the men, and the women are homemakers. The farmers in the three communities utilize both canal-irrigation and dry-farming techniques. Most of the staple food items, such as corn, beans, squash, tomatoes, and chili, are grown in the dry-farming areas, which receive from 6–12 inches of rain during the months of June through September. The rain falls mainly in the form of cloudbursts, and the downpours are often so heavy that young plants are plastered down on the soil and do not survive. The economic position of these families would be much lower if they were not able to utilize a system of irrigation. If attempts to grow crops in the dry-farming areas near the village fail in any one year, the farmers have the assurance of money or credit from the commercial crops. It appears that the normal diet of these villagers is typical, at best, only of other Mexicans in communities with irrigation.

Three methods were used in collecting data, and each encountered difficulties. The first method was to select an informant and obtain his permission to follow him about continuously during his waking hours. Notes were taken as to what he ate during this time, the approximate quantity of the substance consumed, and the hour of the day or night when it was eaten. Notes were also taken on what members of his immediate family ate, but attention was focused on one person at a time. The informant's activities during his waking hours were also noted (walking, standing, running, plowing, cutting alfalfa, grinding corn, talking). There was an attempt to continue this tagging along for three or four days consecutively, but usually the individual informant got weary of the constant companionship and begged off, or found it convenient to do an errand very early on the second or third morning of the observation period. A total of 48 daily diets of individuals was collected in this manner.

A second method was to ask the teachers in the local public schools to have their students write down everything they had eaten the day before. In two of the three communities, I was able to get the fifth and sixth grade classes to cooperate with my project. The teachers took the project under their direction and oversaw the record making. Both the teachers and I went about the room and prompted each student to put down everything he ate from ice cones to the exact number of tortillas. When this task was done, I conducted an "English lesson," using the words and phrases in their diet descriptions as the core of the lesson. The diets of the school children were collected over a two-week period, so that I had a more or less reliable fourteen day diet for each child. During the two-week period, I selected twelve child-informants and visited their homes. While visiting a child's home, I asked other members of his family whether or not he had actually eaten all the items he had listed. I was informed in most cases that the reporting was indeed an actual statement of what the child had eaten the day before. I was aware that Mexican families place high value on supporting members of their immediate family against outsiders regardless of the issue. This accounts for the high correlation of data supplied by the youngster with that supplied by the other members. Yet, my visits to the families indicated my concern over an accurate report of food intake, and I suspect that the subsequent daily reports were more carefully done. I had no difficulty in getting these young informants to take me to their homes. All seemed happy to have a "gringo" in tow and welcomed the opportunity to show off their newly learned English words. The parents were pleased to see and hear their children practice the new words for foods, and often the parents and older siblings would try the new words for *trigo* (wheat) or *azúcar* (sugar). I have included in this analysis the 48 daily diets obtained from the school children.

The third method of obtaining data on daily diets utilized the personnel in a government health clinic in Calipam which served that town and Coxcatlan some four miles away. In this situation, the public health nurse asked the mothers to tell her what they had eaten during the previous day. The responses were written down by the nurse, and this was continued for two weeks for each of the 34 mothers. A government ration of milk was given as part of postnatal care and consumed during the visit to the clinic. However, while it did affect the diet of the mother and her newly arrived child, it was eliminated as a feature in the diet for purposes of analysis because both the clinic and the mothers placed milk in the same category as medicine, which also might be administered during the clinic visit.

The sample of 130 individuals had 85 youngsters below the age of 14 years, of whom 47 were female and 38 male. Of the adults there were 30 males and 15 females. The sample, therefore, had a total of 68 males and 62 females. The weight of the 130 individuals ranged from 50 to 120 pounds for the youngsters and in the adult group from 95 to 210 pounds. The diets of the individuals varied considerably; however, the following is a typical diet:

TABLE 1

TYPICAl DIET

Breakfast	Coffee with sugar; roll-wheat product or 2 tortillas; leftover refried beans, usually with lard, oil, or grease mixed in
Mid Day	Soup or meat broth, high seasoned, with wheat flour noodles; Beans, ½ cup; 3-4 newly cooked tortillas; every third day a small portion of meat; Coffee; Chili in vinegar
Evening meal	Wheat bread with colored sugar on top; beans and tortillas left over from the previous meal; beans mashed and refried
Non-scheduled feeding	Chewing gum, fruit, beer* pulque,* sweetened ice cones.

*Adults only

It is possible that not all individuals or, perhaps, none of these particular 130 individuals actually ate each item on the "typical" diet in a given 24-hour period. However, a typical diet contains 1,433 calories, 43.7 grams protein, and .3951 milligrams calcium (see Table 2).

Another view of daily food consumption is obtained by determining frequency of occurrence of any one item in a daily diet. Charts for each of the major feeding periods are presented below.

It is noteworthy that there is a 95% chance that an

TABLE 2

TYPICAL DIET CONSUMPTIONS

	Calories	Protein grams	Calcium milligrams
Breakfast			
Coffee with sugar	50	0.0	.005
Roll-wheat	95	2.3	.021
Refried beans	130	3.6	.124
	275	5.9	.150
Mid Day			
Soup or meat broth with noodles	125	0.8	.046
Beans ½ cup	115	4.6	.043
3½ tortillas	228	6.5	.140
Meat	111	15.1	.052
Coffee with sugar	50	0.0	.005
	629	27.0	.286
Evening Meal			
Wheat roll with sugar	120	2.3	.024
Beans	115	4.6	.043
2 tortillas	130	3.6	.124
	365	10.5	.191
Other			
Chewing Gum	4	--	--
Fruit	122	1.0	.0080
Alcoholic beverage	36	0.3	.0001
Ice cone	2	0.0	.0000
	164	1.3	.0081
Total of daily intake	1,433	44.7	.6351

individual in our group of 130 people will eat a tortilla for breakfast, and a 96% chance he will eat two tortillas at the

TABLE 3

BREAKFAST

Percentage of chance for	Type of Food
70	Coffee/sugar
50	Sweet or salt roll of wheat
95	One tortilla of corn
35	Beans
40	Milk
30	Chocolate
5	Fruit

MID-DAY MEAL

Percentage of chance for	Type of Food
65	Soup or meat broth with some form of noodles made of wheat
60	Rice cooked in meat broth
80	Chili sauce
96	Two tortillas
80	Beans, ½ cup
20	Meat, 4 oz.
50	Coffee/sugar
30	Coffee with milk and sugar
10	Fruit
5	Goat Cheese
20	Soft drink

EVENING MEAL

Percentage of chance for	Type of Food
70	Beans
30	Soup or meat broth with noodles made of wheat

TABLE 3

Percentage of chance for	Type of Food
40	Chili sauce
35	Hard roll
45	Sugar topped soft roll
70	Coffee/sugar
60	One tortilla
35	One piece of fruit
	NON-SCHEDULED FEEDING
70	Fruit
80	Snow cone or sweetened ice in plastic container or on stick
65	Chewing gum
30	Soft drink
35	Squash seeds
40	Candy (one piece)
65	16 oz. mild alcoholic beverage Pulque, Beer, Tepache (Adults only)
60	6 oz distilled alcoholic beverage-Mescal, Rum, Tequila (Adults only)

mid-day meal. Coffee is ingested by 50% of our sample at both breakfast and at mid-day, whereas chocolate is consumed much less frequently. Tea is not mentioned nor was it observed as a drink among the group of 130, probably because it is expensive and considered a luxury item in all the communities. Therefore, in an overall way, all individuals in this sample eat a corn product at least once a day, all eat some beans, many if not most have coffee with

TABLE 4

NORMAL CANADIAN DIETS

	Weight in lbs	Age	Type of activity	Calories	Protein	Calcium
Children (both sexes)	7-20	0-1		360-900	12-14	0.5
	31	3		1,400	30	0.7
	40	5		1,700	30	0.7
	57	7		2,100	40	1.0
	57	9		2,100	40	1.0
	77	10-12		2,500	50	1.2
Girls	108	13-15		2,600	75	1.2
	120	16-17		2,400	50	1.2
	124	18-19		2,450	50	0.9
Boys	108	13-15		3,100	75	1.2
	136	16-17	Moderate	3,700	55	1.2
	144	18-19	Moderate	3,800	60	0.9
Women	111		Sedentary	1,750	35	0.5
	111		Intense	3,300	35	0.5
	136		Sedentary	2,050	43	0.5
	136		Intense	3,800	43	0.5
Men	144		Sedentary	2,150	46	0.5
	144		Intense	4,000	46	0.5
	176		Sedentary	2,500	55	0.5
	176		Very Intense	5,350	55	0.5

Source: Adapted from *Nutricion Humana.* Organizacion Pan Americana de La Salud, Washington, D.C., 1966, No. 146, p. 154.

sugar at least once a day, and most have a portion of wheat (rolls) once a day. There are many individuals in our group of 130 that do not have meat, milk, or a milk product once a day. The absence of milk or cheese is surprising, since one community is a milk producing village, but the pattern here is to sell the milk to wholesalers from nearby towns for final processing into other milk products. It is later sold at an urban market.

The daily intake of about 1,450 calories seems inadequate in regard to the usual labor done by the people in each of these communities. This is especially apparent if we use the Normal Canadian Diet figures (see Table 4). For example, an adult female of about 110 lbs. needs 1,750 calories a day if she is sedentary and about 3,300 if she is very active. In like manner an adult male of about 145 lbs. needs 2,150 calories if he is sedentary and about 4,000 if he engages in hard work such as plowing or cutting sugar cane.

A list of activities and the utilization of calories on a per hour basis is given above in Table 5, and the additional needs for an 8-hour workday are provided in Table 6. In most observed work or play activities done by the people in the three commercial communities, action was considered "moderate"; therefore, each person needed an additional 500–750 calories per day. Using the Normal Canadian Diet figures for an average man or woman, we arrive at a total need of 2,250 calories for a woman and 2,900 for a man. The comparison of these figures with my data of 1,450 calories per day for an individual indicates that the caloric intake by these Mexican villagers needs to be increased by 800 units for the women and doubled for the men. The same imbalance is observed in the caloric needs of the youngsters. A glance at basic metabolism (Table 7) for young males indicates that the young people in all

TABLE 5

APPROXIMATE ENERGY USE*

Activity	Cal/per hour
Dressing-undressing	33
Sitting in repose	15
Standing at ease	20
Standing at attention	20-25
Walking	130-200
Running	500-930
Singing	37
Reading out loud	20
Washing dishes	59
Ironing	59
Writing	10-20
Thinking	7-8
Working as a carpenter ...	180
Cutting firewood	420
Typing rapidly	16-40
Mining coal	320
Heavy sport playing	980

*For a man 165 lbs. or a woman 130 lbs.

TABLE 6

ADDITIONAL CALORIC NEEDS FOR 8 HR. WORKDAY

Activity	Men	Women
Quiet	225	225
Moderate work	750	500
Heavy work	1,500	1,000
Very heavy work	2,500	

Source: For Tables 5 and 6: Adapted from *Nutricion Humana* Organizacion Pan Americana de la Salud, Washington, D.C., No. 146, p. 32, 1966

TABLE 7

CALORIC NEEDS OF YOUNG MALES PER DAY

Age	Basic Metabolism	Quiet	Active	Very Active
0	200			
1	500	750		
2	800	1,200	1,600	2,350
4	900	1,400	1,860	2,800
6	1,100	1,600	2,160	3,230
8	1,200	1,800	2,400	3,630
10	1,300	2,000	2,640	3,950
12	1,440	2,130	2,870	4,300
14	1,470	2,200	2,950	4,400
15	1,550	2,300	3,100	4,620

Source: Modified from original data: G. Lusk, Requirements for Nutrition. JAMA Vol. 70:821 - 1918.

three of the Mexican villages obtain barely enough calories to maintain basic metabolism.

An additional view can be gotten from the general needs a person has to have to live adequately in a temperate climate. These are presented in Table 8, where we note again that 1,450 calories per day is very low and seemingly insufficient to maintain a proper level of activity.

Obviously something is amiss. The people studied did plow, sew, talk, cut wood, run, and walk. They were all active and busy with a number of tasks many hours of the day. There are at least two sources of error. First, the Normal Canadian Diet figures may be too high and may need to be adjusted downward. Second, the data I have collected may be faulty. I suspect both situations are in need of re-evaluation, and efforts should be directed towards resolving the issues raised. There are many problems involved in getting precise field data. In Mexican villages,

TABLE 8

CALORIC NEEDS PER DAY/TEMPERATE CLIMATE

Age	Men	Women
20-30	3,200	2,300
30-40	3,104	2,231
40-50	3,008	2,162
50-60	2,768	1,990
60-70	2,528	1,817
70	2,208	1,587

Source: Adapted from *Nutricion Humana* Organizacion Pan Americana de la Salud, Washington, D.C., No. 146, p. 35, 1966.

one cannot collect feces with any safety (accusations of practicing witchcraft would immediately result); therefore, except in highly structured experimental situations, residue examination would be impossible. Counting and weighing food brought into a home or hearth is possible, but the fact that almost all individuals eat "snacks" while moving about makes the hearth method by itself inaccurate. The "tag-along" method used in the collection of this data is very difficult to sustain over a long enough period of time for it to be generally valid as a measure. The "tag-along" method necessitates the use of a large number of personnel which is not generally available. It appears that a combination of measuring what comes into a home for consumption and the tag-along method would be the most productive in getting accurate data on daily diets. Research activity of this sort would mean that the investigator(s) needs to live with a family and tag-along as a member of that group as the individuals go about daily tasks. A six to eight month period should be long enough to determine the general eating patterns of a family numbering from six to sixteen members. The data acquired in this manner would be more realistic in many ways, for within a family eating pattern certain high ranking adults (fathers and elder sons) get first choice of the things to eat, and usually a Mexican family has special preferences toward certain "hot" versus "cold" foods which are not necessarily community-wide. This live-in activity is normal for ethnographers, and all that is suggested is that there be special attention focused on dietary activities of the people being studied. It is safe to assume that most ethnographers already have such material in their field notes, and perhaps it can be organized into an ethnographic bank for refinement and publication. Data of this sort could then be used to revise the normal caloric needs of various populations of people who are practicing different ways of life in both similar and differing ecological situations. These new diet evaluations could then be used in combination with food getting practices or producton data, and, thereby, establish the degree of surplus that the various subsistence systems actually produce. This method is basically a way to get data on energy input-output in human populations. It is co-joined with the hope that in the future field workers will get reliable data on human daily diets so that the input end of the energy system can be determined. The surplus that is needed to create or maintain cultural activities such as monument building (pyramids, warships, irrigation systems, or town plazas) is still grossly estimated and will continue to be only a general guess until the input end of the continuum is known for cultures of varied ecological settings and complexities.

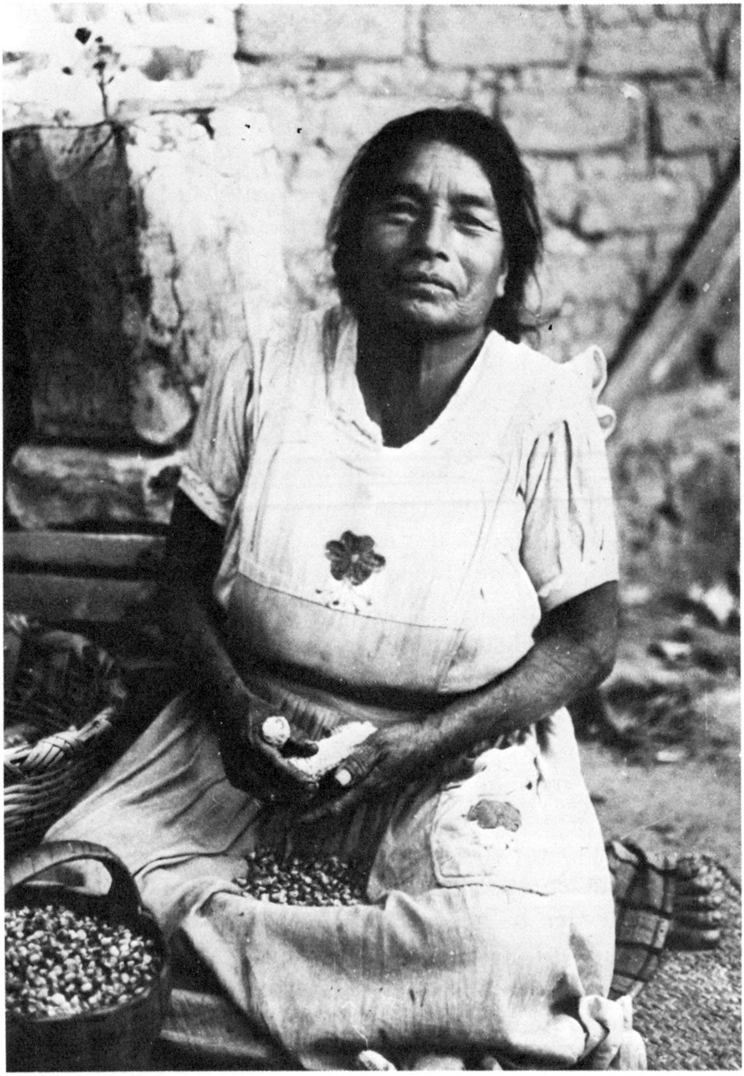

Shelling dry corn by Zapotec villager in Matatlan, Oaxaca. Shelled corn is soaked in lime-water over-night, then ground up to make tortillas. (1968)

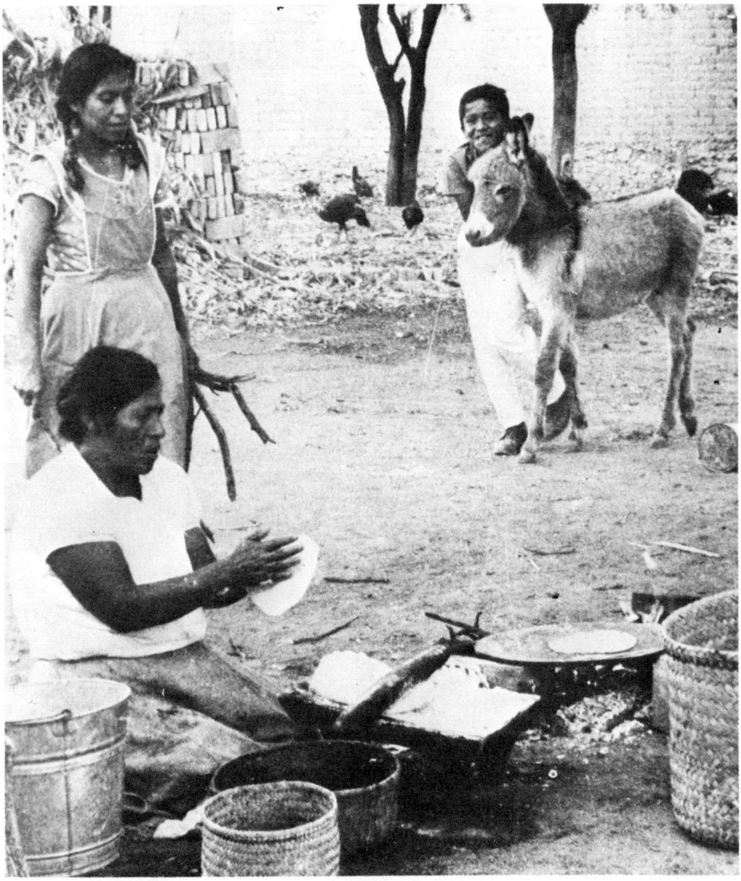

Tortilla making in Chapulco, Puebla. Corn kernels ground up on the *metate* with the *mano* (next to the knees of the woman patting out the tortilla), then shaped into thin moist disk and cooked on the *comal* over the fire. (1966)

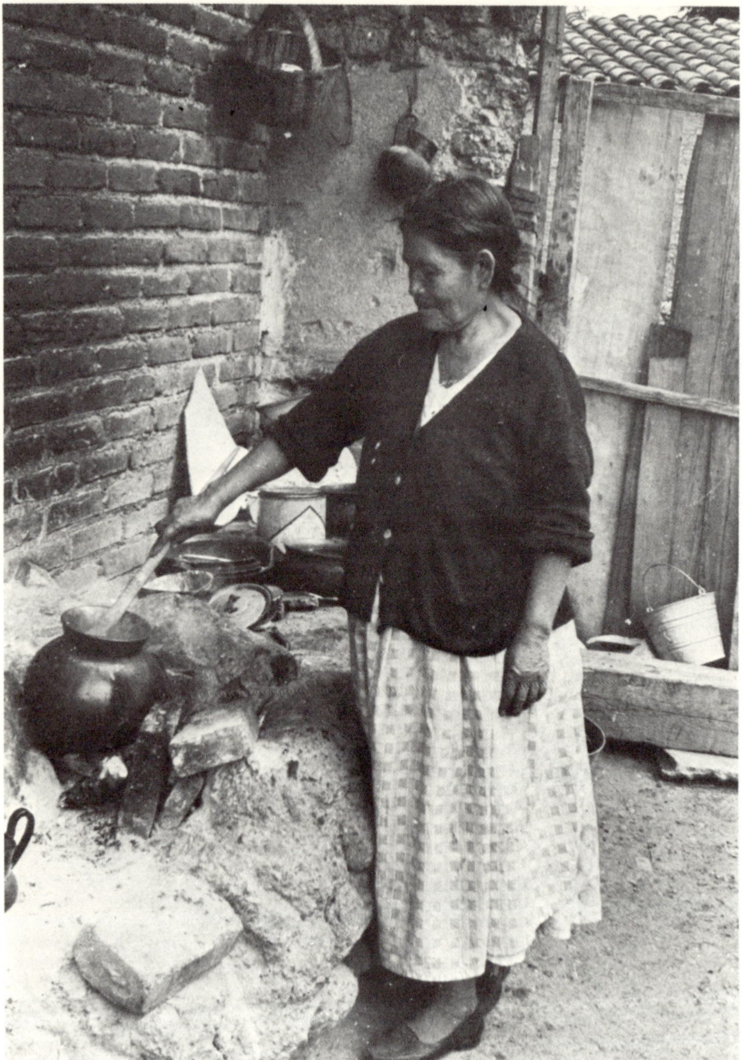

Beans being stirred by elderly matron in San Gabriel Etla, Oaxaca. This cooking area is used only in the summer time. Winter cooking is done indoors. (1969)

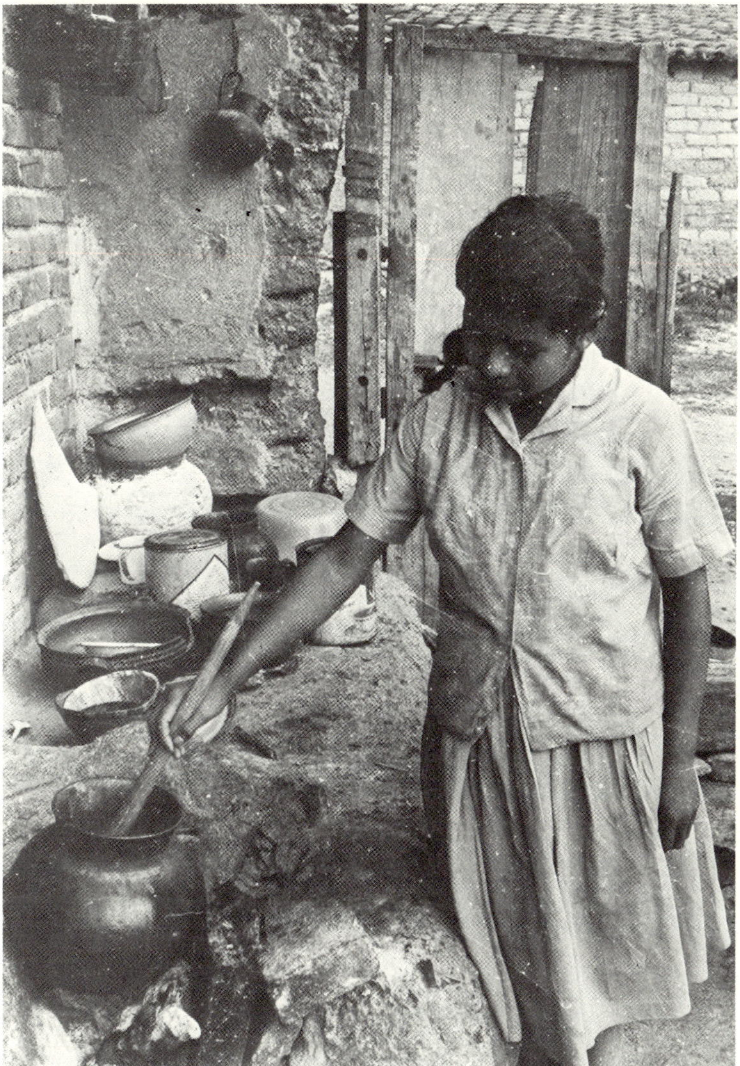

Beans being stirred by youngster in San Gabriel Etla, Oaxaca. This cooking area is used only in the summer time. Winter cooking is done indoors. (1969)

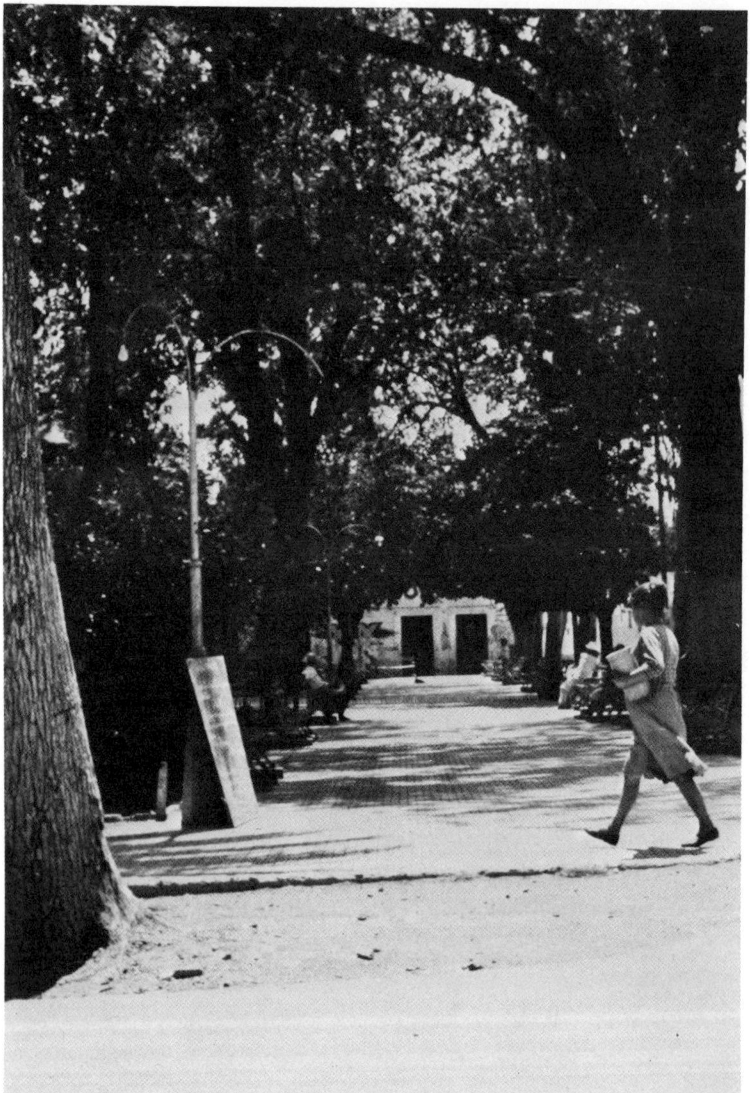

Young matron striding through central plaza in Coxcatlan, Puebla. (1964)

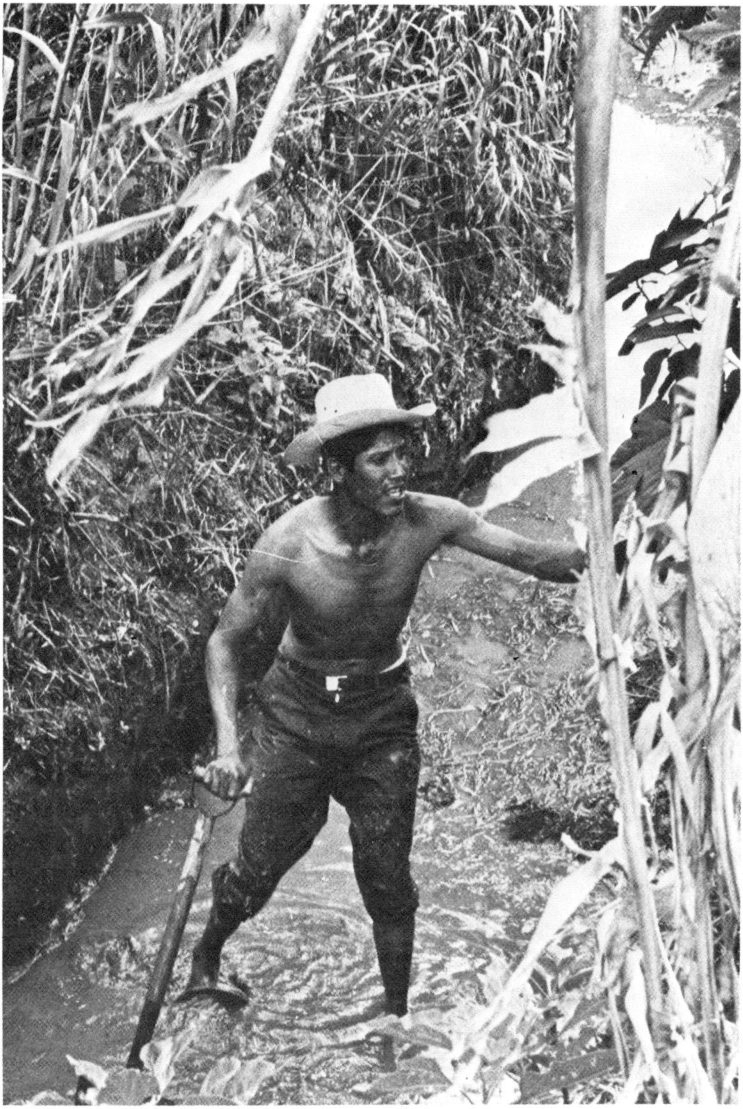

Irrigation canal being cleaned of sediment by young farmer in Coxcatlan, Puebla. (1964)

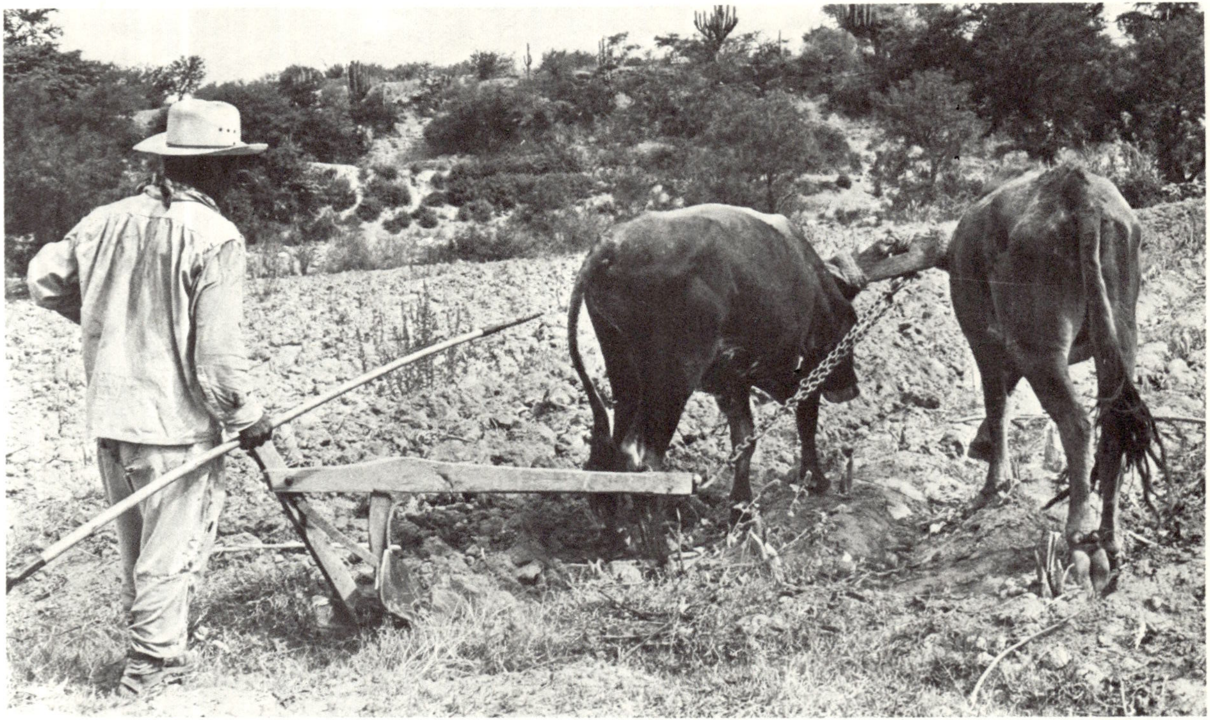

Field being prepared for crops near Coxcatlan, Puebla. (1964)

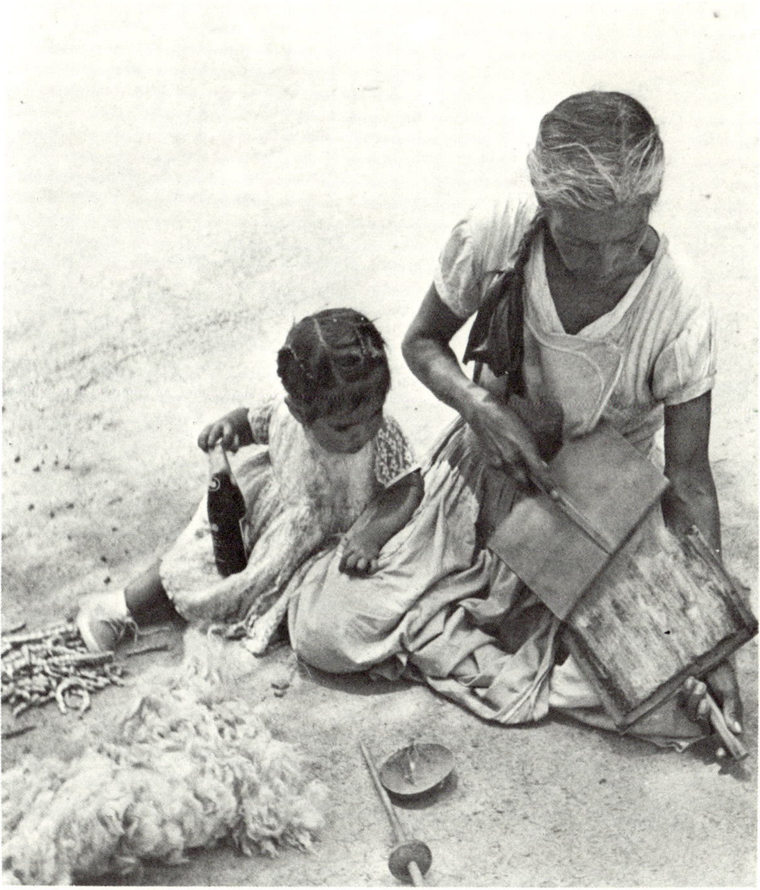

Grandmother carding wool as grand-daughter watches and holds carbonated soft-drink which is being shared in Mitla, Oaxaca. (1968)

Lawrence Kaplan

ETHNOBOTANICAL AND NUTRITIONAL FACTORS IN THE DOMESTICATION OF AMERICAN BEANS

The principal nutritional significance of *Phaseolus* beans has probably always been derived from the use of the dry seeds as a source of vegetable protein. Several species, particularly *Phaseolus vulgaris,* supply edible immature pods and seeds—that is, snapbeans—but, because of their high water content at this stage (about 89%), they do not function as an important dietary protein. On a dry weight basis, the protein content of the immature pod and beans together totals about 10%; that of mature seeds, however, may be anywhere from 22% to 40%.

The close relationship between beans and corn in the indigenous diet of the populous cultures of Mesoamerica and the Andean region is, like other traditional dietary combinations, no accident. Quantitative chemical analyses of corn and beans as used in the diets of contemporary Yucatecan Indians show complementation between the principal corn protein, zein, and the alpha and beta globulins of black beans. Reports of experimental nutritional studies indicate that where zein is the principal protein in the diet of a monogastric animal, lysine is the limiting amino acid that must be made up from another source.

Beans, with a high lysine content compared to that of corn, supply this amino acid, and a dietary protein combination of high biological value is achieved. Although not particularly high in tryptophane, beans do appear to supply enough of this amino acid to supplement the tryptophane derived from corn. Because tryptophane acts as a precursor for the formation of niacine (when tryptophane is in excess of the dietary requirement (Bressani *et al.*, 1955), the amount of tryptophane in a corn-and-beans diet successfully replaces the niacine lost in the preparation of corn tortillas. In Guatemalan diets, where corn consumption may be 500 grams per day and bean consumption may be 75 grams per day, the total tryptophane taken in is likely to be in excess of that required for protein building. Some of this may be converted, or, at least, is available for conversion to niacine. Excess tryptophane, plus the niacine present in beans, may account for the absence of pellagra in the corn-bean consuming areas of Central America and Mexico, according to reports of Scrimshaw, Harris, Bressani, and others associated with I.N.C.A.P. In some geographic areas, insufficient consumption of corn and beans or, perhaps, local environmental factors or local varieties of corn and beans result in deficiencies of critical amino acids; and, therefore, a dietary protein of adequate biological value is not achieved.

Protein shortage resulting in clinical symptoms has, of course, been long and widely noted in some predominantly Indian areas of Latin America. The defective feeding of children from one to four years of age that produces symptoms now referred to as kwashiokor is world-wide. This was recognized and reported in 1903 in Yucatan as *culebrilla* (Scrimshaw & Behar, 1959). It is now widely known that protein requirements vary and that proteins adequate in amount and quality for adult males may be inadequate for some protein-sensitive members of a population, such as recently weaned children and lactating mothers (Altschul, 1962).

Beans of different varieties and even of different *Phaseolus* species are moderately high in lysine and tryptophane. Corn varies considerably in total proteins as do beans, but corn is always deficient in lysine and tryptophane (Block & Weiss, 1956). Because amino acid complementation exists in many different combinations of corn varieties and bean varieties and species, in early prehistoric agricultural times a kind of universal flexibility in the adaptation of these dietary components to human requirements resulted. It is now clear that corn and beans were not domesticated simultaneously nor did they necessarily diffuse together in some areas—for example, Tamaulipas (Kaplan & MacNeish, 1960) and coastal Peru (Towle, 1961). However, whenever these two food crops met, an immediate adaptive combination favored by human selections was formed.

The evolution of the human diet is marked perhaps to a greater extent by synergistic combinations than by small increments in the food value of individual nutrient sources. Because the nutritional insufficiency of plant seed proteins is the result of limiting amino acids rather than low total protein content, raising the total protein content would not make it more effective in the diet. As a matter of fact, according to I.N.C.A.P. studies, since zein is the fraction of poorest quality in terms of balance of amino acids in corn, the loss of zein in the preparation of tortillas probably results in improving total effectiveness of corn proteins although the total corn protein is reduced.

The answer to the problem of lysine as the limiting amino acid in corn has been found in the supplementation of corn with beans rather than through changes in the total proteins of corn or in the array of the amino acids of corn during the evolution of indigenous American nutrition.

How did such a useful combination come about? Doubtless, repeated sampling of the available plant resources resulted in the combination. Seasonality, ecological factors, compatibility with other crops, and ongoing ways of human life were factors, as well as were the nutrients, in determining the adoption of supplementary crops. Sampling the vegetation over a period of perhaps 1,400 to 3,000 years prior to the establishment of corn and bean agriculture, roughly 6,000 years ago in Middle America, was evidently sufficient to establish this combination. Given sufficient time, a comparable biota, and similar human practices, the same plants would probably be domesticated all over again.

Factors leading toward the domestication of plants, particularly those based on nutritional sampling and selection, remain open more to speculation than to data referral. Later, I will try to suggest some of the data that must be accumulated in order to reduce the speculative content.

Surprisingly, few quantitative studies of normal Middle American Indian diets have been made. The difficulty in obtaining such information free of gross error and the necessity of long-term observation have been noted by various field workers. Nevertheless, it has been necessary to make quantitative estimates of food intake, especially where programs for the correction of nutritional deficiencies have been initiated. Archaeological studies on nutrition are also few in number and include a high percentage of error. Human nutrition as a science is no less uncertain in many respects, at least to the view of an outsider, than are the surveys of food intake. That which constitutes a normal or optimum protein requirement depends on variables such as size, sex, stage of growth, lactation, physical activity, balance of diet, and inherited factors affecting protein utilization, which certainly differs among individuals and may differ among human biological populations.

The absence of reliable data on these variables makes any discussion of the sort attempted here highly speculative. Hopefully, speculation will stimulate the gathering of data.

MacNeish and his co-workers have attempted to reconstruct an ancient diet qualitatively and quantitatively. The probability of gross error is inevitably great but, with care, can be recognized. In the Tehuacan Valley, over a period beginning about 9,000 years ago and ending at the time of the Spanish Conquest, an overall trend to reduce the hunted meat component of the diet from 60% to 17% took place. Meat was increasingly replaced by cultivated plants, and these showed a steady increase in relation to edible wild plants. In the process of change from a hunting and gathering economy to one based on plant husbandry, the measurable portion of corn in the diet steadily rose. It accounted, eventually, for most of the plant foot eaten. In the same period, the estimated quantities of beans increased, but the error here must be extremely high since beans are unlikely to produce measurable remains no matter how abundant they are. For example, in contemporary Indian cultures, bushbeans are threshed in the fields where pods and plants are simply discarded. Dry mature polebeans are frequently stripped of the seeds and left on the vines. An analysis of the Tehuacan figures suggests that in Venta Salada times (ca. AD 700 to 1540) about 90% of the diet from cultivated plants was corn; since cultivated plants constituted 75% of the total diet, corn made up about 67% of the total diet. The same figures suggest that beans made up only 1/100 of 1% of the corn intake. This looks a bit low.

Another view of paleonutrition might result from considering the corn-bean ratio to be similar to that which obtains at present in some Indian cultures. According to the I.N.C.A.P. figures, some 500 grams of corn are consumed per day by adult males in the Guatemalan highlands. This amount yields about 80% of the calories and 70% of the protein intake, although the protein content of corn varies considerably. The protein actually derived from such corn intake varies from about 35 to 56 grams per day. According to I.N.C.A.P. figures (Bressani *et al.*, 1955) bean (*P. vulgaris*) consumption in rural Central America varies from 30 to 120 grams daily. This range corresponds with my observations in rural Mexico. Therefore, the consumption of beans should, at minimum, be 6% that of corn and may rise to 24% that of corn.

In Tehuacan, the relatively high proportion of meat estimated in the diet, 17% in Venta Salada times, would appear to support this seeming rarity of beans. Remembering that the meat component of the Tehuacan diet was estimated at 65% in early times, if these figures are accepted, the cultivation of beans as a protein source appears unlikely. Although the estimates of meat consumption may be high and the estimates of bean consumption may be low, it is clear that a good deal of meat was consumed, and the importance of beans as a protein food may have been correspondingly less.

Although estimating quantities of food intake is one approach to the study of paleonutrition, it is much in need of refined techniques. Another approach to the study of ancient human nutrition is to add an estimate of the nutrient quality to the estimate of total quantity of dietary elements. I noted earlier that both beans and corn vary greatly in total protein as a result of genetic and environmental influences, the array of amino acids varies somewhat, and the amino acid levels in corn and beans tend to be complementary. It is less well known that the protein content of beans varies inversely to the seed size. The broad screening data of Earle and Jones (1962), which they presented in tabular form, are presented here in graphic form (Fig. 1). The strong inverse correlation between size and protein content is obvious. One of the overall trends in the domestication of beans is increase in seed size (Kaplan, 1965). Although a complete sequence from wild *P. vulgaris* to cultivated *P. vulgaris* is unknown, we do have some indication as to how recently small-seeded wild beans were in use and when large-seeded domesticates became available.

In the Tehuacan Valley, domesticated *vulgaris* beans were present 7,000 years ago with no evidence of the use of small-seeded wild beans. The ongoing excavations near Mitla, Oaxaca, disclose that small wild beans were utilized 9,000 years ago. The highly twisted pods support the judgment that these were, indeed, wild beans. The identity of these seeds has not yet been established, but the structure of the meristematic embryo does not conform to the *vulgaris* pattern. These wild seeds have not yet been analyzed for protein content, but we may suppose that the protein content is high, because analyses of modern, small-seeded, wild beans show a high protein content. The yield of a field crop is, of course, a factor influencing its feasibility as a source of protein. We know little about the relationship between seed size, yield, total protein, and proportions of amino acids among cultivated varieties. We know absolutely nothing about these parameters in wild beans. By inference, however, we are probably safe in thinking that the small-seeded wild *P. vulgaris* relatives had higher protein levels than large-seeded domesticated beans. Therefore, in the case of the early Oaxaca cultures, small wild beans were abundant 9,000 years ago and continued in the record until 1,000 years ago. Corn was introduced or domesticated later than beans, and the remains are poorly preserved. No data are yet available on meat. Estimates of food resources obtained from wild plants versus cultivated plants and species or varietal breakdowns of

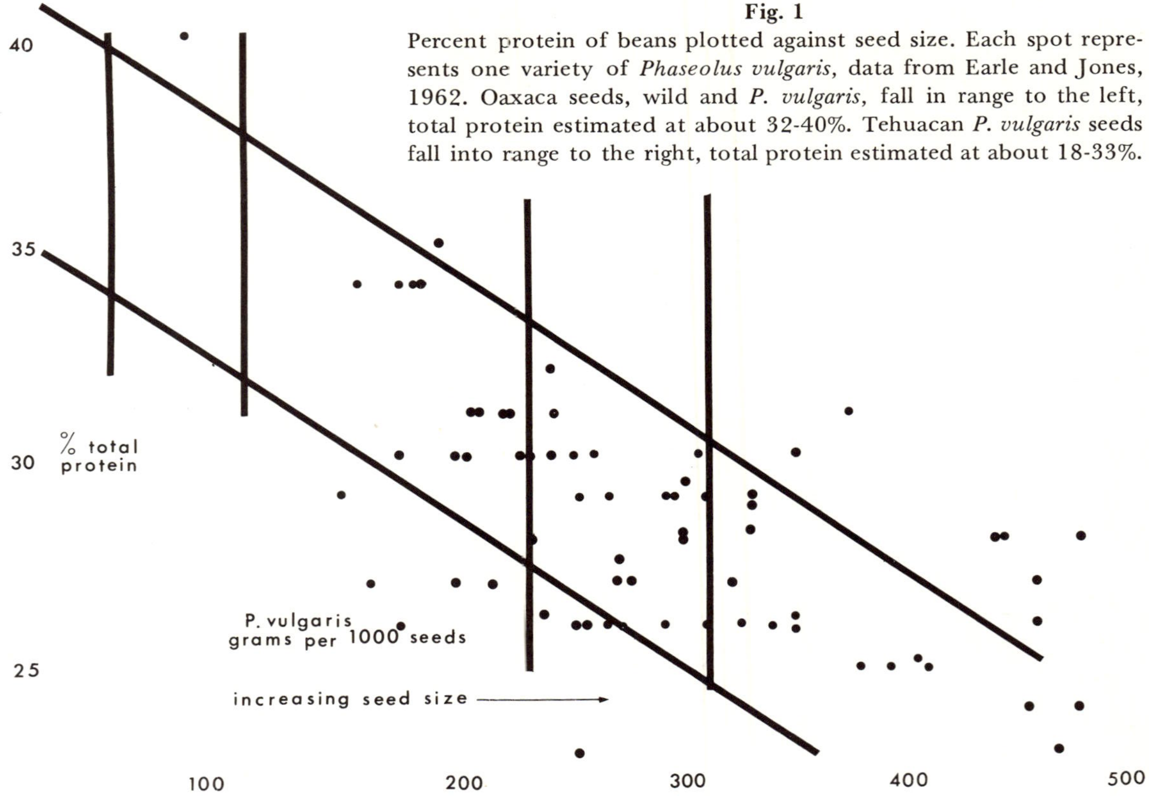

Fig. 1

Percent protein of beans plotted against seed size. Each spot represents one variety of *Phaseolus vulgaris*, data from Earle and Jones, 1962. Oaxaca seeds, wild and *P. vulgaris*, fall in range to the left, total protein estimated at about 32-40%. Tehuacan *P. vulgaris* seeds fall into range to the right, total protein estimated at about 18-33%.

these are not yet available. Referring to Figure 1, from which we can extrapolate protein content versus seed size for the early beans, it is strikingly evident that the beans used in the valley of Oaxaca were far higher in protein content than those used at the same periods in the Tehuacan Valley. Furthermore, they were far higher in protein than beans that were introduced later, and the small-seeded beans continued to be used in the Oaxaca Valley in historic times despite the fact that, in prehistoric times, the larger-seeded, presumably higher yielding beans were available either from Tehuacan or other areas. These preliminary observations suggest that near Mitla in the Oaxaca Valley, in contrast to the Tehuacan Valley, meat was scarce and protein was derived largely from plant sources. Small-seeded wild beans and, later, the relatively small-seeded bean cultivars provided the main source of protein. Here we see two areas roughly comparable in time and roughly comparable in environment, yet differing markedly in the utilization of beans in the diet. Parenthetically, we might ask, when we speak of the diet, "Whose diet?". That is, if meat were available, would it be available to everyone—men, women, children, captives, slaves?

Much is wanting in the data that are available; but it is clear, even at this point, that a differential selection was operating that favored large-seeded, low protein beans in Tehuacan and relatively small-seeded, high protein beans in Oaxaca. The peoples of these valleys were not isolated. They traded other materials; therefore, the differences in their bean varieties cannot be laid to isolation nor to the unavailability of other bean varieties. I would again suggest that we pay more attention to nutrient value in our consideration of factors that set the evolutionary stage for domestication and agriculture.

Now, what about beans in the protein-short, overpopulated, and economically depressed areas of the world? N. W. Pirie (1969), in a provocative advocacy of biochemical engineering and the development of novel protein sources, dismisses beans and other well-known traditional protein resources, because these will be used effectively without special programs and special effort. However, it might be profitable for nutritional biochemists, as well as the plant taxonomists and ethnobotanists, to investigate more closely some of our traditional resources. In the case of beans, we may conclude that traditional utilization and production are all wrong. We may really want low yields of primitive, small-seeded beans to act as supplements in diets low in animal proteins. Continuing interdisciplinary studies of prehistoric and contemporary primitive, but long adapted, subsistence may suggest that there are great reservoirs of useful, nutritional novelty in the extant varieties of beans and other ancient domesticates.

REFERENCES

Altschul, Aaron M. 1962. "Seed protein and world food problems." *Econ. Bot.* 16: 2-13.

Block, Richard J., and Weiss, Kathryn W. 1956. *Amino Acid Handbook.* Charles C. Thomas, Springfield, Illinois.

Bressani, R. W., Marcucci, E., Robles, C. Enrique, and Scrimshaw, N. S. 1955. *"Valor Nutritivo de los frijoles Centroamericanos." Boletin de la Officina Sanitaria Panamericana Publicaciones del Instituto de Nutricion de Centroamerica y Panama* (INCAP). Suppl. 2: 201-206. (Originally published in *Food Research* 19: 263-268. Nutritive value of Central American Beans. I. INCAP I 15. 1954).

Earle, F. R., and Jones, Quentin. 1962. "Analysis of Seed Samples from 113 Plant Families." *Econ. Bot.* 16 (4): 221-250.

Kaplan, L., and MacNeish, R. S. 1960. "Prehistoric bean remains from caves in the Ocampo region of Tamaulipas, Mexico." *Bot. Mus. Leafl.* Harvard University 19 (2): 33-56.

Kaplan, L. 1965. "Archaeology and Domestication in American Phaseolus (Beans)." *Econ. Bot.* 19 (4): 358-368.

MacNeish, R. S., et al. 1967. *The Prehistory of the Tehuacan Valley.* Vol. 1. Environment and Subsistence. University of Texas Press.

Pirie, N. W. 1969. *Food Resources* Pelican - Penguin.

Scrimshaw, N. S., and Behar, M. 1959. "World wide occurrence of protein malnutrition." *Fed. Proc.* 18: 82-87.

Towle, Margaret A. 1961. *The ethnobotany of Pre-Columbian Peru.* Viking Fund Publications in Anthropology, No. 30. Wenner Gren Foundation for Archaeological Research, Inc., New York.

Jacques Barrau
(Translated by Roda and Colin Roberts)

THE OCEANIANS AND THEIR FOOD PLANTS

(A Sketch of Nutritional Ethnobotany of the Tropical Pacific Islands)

Ethnobotany is such a young discipline that it still must find its own definition, as well as establish whether it belongs among the natural sciences or the humanities, or somewhere between. This has provoked and continues to provoke some rather useless discussions. Because this essay needs a framework, however, I will choose to define ethnobotany according to the broad quasi-etymological sense of the term, understanding it simply as the study of the relations between peoples and the plant world, where the latter refers only to food plants, wild or cultivated.

Like other plant species with economic interest, food plants are too often scorned by botanists. It goes without saying, however, that they evoke a definite interest and are of primary importance; there is hardly a part of the world whose history is not rich in examples of dramas, of upsets, or of progress caused by the accidental failure of a basic food culture or the introduction, discovery, or domestication of a food plant offering new resources.

This symposium will permit us to make a rapid assessment of our knowledge about the role of plants of alimentary interest in tropical Oceania, where *Oceania* has the initial definition given to it by Dumont d'Urville (1832): in his eyes, we remember, it extended from the Sunda Islands to far eastern Polynesia, through the two arcs that comprise Micronesia and Melanesia. This is an old definition and certainly a disputable one, but it is a practical one for the purpose of this essay, since, speaking only of the useful plants with ancient existence in this part of the world, the relationship of the economic flora from the western to the eastern Pacific is obvious. In fact, the area of this study is the Malay-Oceanian sphere whose agrobotanical and ethnobotanical interest I have mentioned elsewhere (Barrau, 1966). Doubtless, the plants and men of Melanesia, Micronesia, and Polynesia will be the most often referred to here. Nevertheless, it is impossible to treat them without speaking about the vast lands further west, since we are, in fact, in the immense Indo-Oceania area defined by Haudricourt and Hedin (1943) in their basic study on man and cultivated plants.

For the study of ethnobotany, this part of the world constitutes an area of fruitful research, because of its ecological and cultural diversity, its wealth of plant life, and the discovery there of food economies which, without doubt, bear witness to very old forms of man's use of plants and of his adaptation to the natural environment.

Throughout its long history, Oceania most certainly witnessed modification in its economic flora as its inhabitants improved their techniques, as they adapted to new environments, and as new migrations of men arrived with ideas, plants, and new methods. These changes have continued to the present and are still going on; the development of commercial crops during the colonial period was an example; another is the upheavals in food production caused in certain islands by the changeover, at times swift and always difficult, from a food economy to a monetary economy. In the area of man's nourishment, such periods of evolution or revolution have given rise (and continue to give rise) to biological, economic, and social problems. This is the inevitable result, considering that plants play such an important part in the economic and social life of human groups. In the overall area of Oceania, it should be remembered, man gets most of his food from plants which he either gathers wild or cultivates, and whose products often account for more than 80% of the foodstuffs traditionally consumed. Gathering and cultivation control, or controlled, the rhythm of the social life of Oceania, which was characterized and is still much characterized by agrarian rites.

In order to better understand the nutritional ethnobotany of Oceania, it might be useful to point out a contrast that is clearly fundamental: west of the Wallace line from Amboina to the Malay Peninsula, a cereal food economy based on rice, *Oryza sativa* L., and on other edible gramineous seeds dominates. Both in olden times and recently, the latter have had an importance which they have maintained in some places; such is the case of millet, *Setaria italica*(L.) Beauv. or of the *adlay* or Job's-tears, *Coix lacryma-jobi L.*

East of the Wallace line, from New Guinea through Micronesia and Polynesia to Easter Island, the dominant food economy is based on the cultivation of taro, *Colocasia esculenta* (L.) Schott, yams (*Dioscorea* spp.), breadfruit, *Artocarpus altilis* (Parkinson) Fosberg, bananas, etc . . . all perennial plants which are propagated by vegetative means and which provide man with tubers or starchy fruits. It may be mentioned too that, in this part of Oceania, wild harvesting still feeds man, for example, in the swamp forest of sago-palm (*Metroxylon* spp.) of the lowlands of New Guinea, where starch extracted from the stems of these palm trees is the basic food.

This contrast between systems of food economy based on cereals and those based on starchy perennials has been recognized since Rumphius (1750:346) made note of it during the seventeenth century in his *Herbarium Amboinense.* It must be added that such a distinction is not without exception, because the tubers and starchy fruits just mentioned, and some others of the same categories, have played and continue to play a definite part in the nourishment of the Sunda Islands and of tropical or subtropical Asia—that is, where the cereals are the dominating element.

There are, besides, very localized cases where rice, millet, taro, yams, etc., are cultivated in equal, or almost equal, quantities, although separately; for example, the Botel Tobago Islands (Kano and Segawa, 1956).

As a general rule, however, no cereals were found east of the Wallace line during the pre-European era; the limits of rice cultivation were at that time Amboinia in the south and the Marianas Islands in the north, where the discoverers of the sixteenth century noted its presence; rice was being cultivated there mainly for the preparation of a fermented drink.

Practically all of the starchy perennial plants which are propagated vegetatively, and which were cultivated in Melanesia, Micronesia, and Polynesia before the arrival of the Europeans, originate from the Indo-Malayan center of origin of cultivated plants, defined by Vavilov (1951), which was spread to the large islands of western Melanesia and to the westermost islands of Micronesia (Barrau, 1962).

From this vast center come the taro, *Colocasia,* and other nourishing Araceae of the genera *Alocasia, Amor-*

phophallus and *Cyrtosperma;* the various yams (*Dioscorea* spp.), whose numbers of species cultivated, or only used, decrease from west to east; the principal bananas, breadfruit, etc. As brief evidence of the extension of Vavilov's Indo-Malayan center to Melanesia and Micronesia, we might remember that the *fehi* banana, *Musa troglodytarum* L., has its origin in New Guinea and the neighboring islands (MacDaniels, 1947; Simmonds, 1959); that the sugar cane, *Saccharum officinarum* L., also began in New Guinea (Artschwager and Brandes, 1958; Warner, 1962); and that the wild parents of the cultivated breadfruit grow in New Guinea and in the Marianas Islands (Barrau, 1959).

The complex of cultivated food plants of the Oceanians, therefore, originates principally in the western part of the region, and the types of archaic food horticulture with which this complex is associated were probably invented at the end of the Pleistocene era (cf. Golson, 1968). This complex advanced toward the east, accompanying the voluntary or accidental migrations of the men who inhabited the islands of the Great Sea.

In this progression towards the rising sun, some plants did not survive the voyage or the landings at all, or did not follow the men all the way to their easternmost discoveries and explorations, or else their use was discontinued because other species were preferred. Thus, the economic flora of the Malay-Oceanian area diminishes as one goes eastward. However, this reduction is often compensated for by refinement and diversification of cultivated plants in the islands farthest from the centers of origin of these plants; thus, the number of clones of the *fehi* banana increases from Melanesia to eastern Polynesia, and the greatest number of cultivated varieties of breadfruit are found in eastern Polynesia (Wilder, 1928; Barrau, 1959).

All this shows quite well that the true domestication of

a plant has often had to be accompanied by movement away from the original habitat; in the same way, improvement of a plant by man and diversification brought about by empirical selection were proportionately more active as the plant food sources were less numerous. The gatherer who has access to a wide variety of wild food plants will hardly be selective, any more than he would need to set about intensive domestication or attempts at cultivation. This seems to be so true that one wonders if the old legend of the Garden of Eden had its origin, in fact, in the longing memory of a happy age when men found all the food they needed in a rich vegetation that they exploited by gathering! To repeat a phrase from Sahlins (1968), the gatherers may have constituted the first affluent society!

This wild harvest is still practiced in New Guinea where it sometimes provides the greater part of the plant foods; such is the case in the marshy *Metroxylon,* sago-palm, forests. Often, even when there is gardening for food, the forest also contributes an appreciable amount to the diet, and this is still apparent in New Guinea (Blackwood, 1940).

Since we are discussing wild gathering, it may be interesting to note here that there could be found in pre-European Oceania all the forms of transition between wild gathering and the advanced stages of cultivation, including those involving a profound change in the cultural environment due to irrigation, drainage, the use of compost, of plants which reestablish the soil, etc. (Barrau, 1962). This helps make Oceania one of the most interesting areas available for research in ethnobotany. In addition, we find food plants in all the various stages of domestication in this part of the world (Barrau, 1967).

We saw above that the bringing in of food plants played an important role in early Oceania, at a time when the navigators of the distant past carried the plants they needed for food from island to island. Almost all the plants came from the large islands in the west, as has already been mentioned, but there are exceptions: the sweet potato, *Ipomoea batatas* (L.) Lamk., which, until further evidence is produced, can be said to come from the American tropics (Conklin, 1963; Nishiyama, 1963; Yen, 1963)—and it is certainly of no use to reopen that debate here. It is worth remarking, however, that the importation of this plant to certain parts of Oceania must have caused quite revolutionary economic and social changes. This was clearly the case in New Guinea, where this member of the Convolvulaceae enabled man's settlement and his proliferation in the highlands of this large island where the other basic food plants characteristic of Oceania, the starchy perennials, could not prosper (Watson, 1964).

Ancient Oceania was certainly the scene of other upheavals related to such introductions of food plants and to other changes in its vegetal complex brought about under similar conditions. The use of the cultivation of certain food plants, thus, was discontinued because more productive or more easily usable species became available. This explains the existence in places of food plants which have been almost forgotten and which truly bear witness to the past (Barrau, 1965). The cordyline, *Cordyline fruticosa* (L.) A. Chev., or *Pueraria lobata* (Wil d.) Ohwi are good examples; so too is the *purao* with edible bark, *Hibiscus tiliaceus* L., still cultivated today in New Caledonia. Such plants have the interesting characteristic of multiple use; for instance, the three species just mentioned are both food plants and fiber plants. This would seem to confirm Sauer's (1952) hypothesis, that fishing and the domestication of plants went hand in hand at the dawn of the Malay Oceanian civilizations; hence the importance in ancient days of fibrous plants which provided necessary materials for the fabrication of primitive fishing and navigation gear. The same author, as you know, insists on the probably early existence of the propagation by vegetative means of perennial plants, at the very beginnings of agriculture in this part of the humid tropics. This seems to be indicated by the archaeological research of Lathrap (1965) in America and Chang (1968) in Southeast Asia.

One might therefore imagine that the Oceanian group first experienced a food economy based on perennial starchy plants which, while they were being domesticated and adapted to cultivation, were propagated by vegetative means.

Later may have come the cereals, *Coix, Setaria* and *Oryza;* and the cultivated flora of old Oceania found refuge in New Guinea and the islands of Melanesia, Micronesia, and Polynesia.

This would explain why some perennial tuberous plants, such as the taro, *Colocasia,* are today still planted ritually by the rice growers of Indo-Malaysia and Asia, as though these people wished to perpetuate in this way the memory of pre-cereal food systems that have disappeared, but which once permitted their ancient ancestors to live, by means of the cultivation of starchy foods propagated by cuttings. What still must be understood is why the cereals became dominant: in food economy, perennials with starchy tubers, like the taro or yam, are of greater interest than cereals; they are easier to cultivate and more readily usable; besides, their yield in food is superior to rice, to take just this cereal as an example, using it for this comparison in terms of its yield before modern agronomic science resulted in its recent improvements.

It is difficult to understand, therefore, what could have induced the tuber gardeners to become rice farmers. This passage from the *hortus* to the *ager*—from garden to field—from individual, friendly care (Haudricourt, 1964) of food plants grown in the garden to mass production in fields, amounts to a veritable revolution. Certainly, rice in its traditional forms of cultivation in Indo–Malaysia was and still is the object of an almost horticultural method (transplanting, harvesting panicle by panicle), and this may be another vestige of cultural traditions related to habits acquired in ancient times from the growing of starchy perennial plants in gardens. However, rice is quite different from these starchy plants; it absolutely must be harvested when mature; its grains, to be edible, must undergo a relatively complex treatment; they must be preserved with care, and this is by no means always easily done in a tropical region. For growers and eaters of tubers, these are clear disadvantages, and this further explains the many failures that the European agronomists suffered when, during the colonial period, they tried to impose the cultivation of rice on Melanesians, traditionally yam and taro gardners. We might take note of this obstinacy on the part of the colonial agronomists in wanting to impose the cultivation of rice on all the inhabitants of the tropics; in their opinion, there definitely could be no civilization or progress possible without cereal, because cereals lend themselves better than tubers to trade.

This last characteristic of cereals played a role, too, in the ancient implanting of millet, and especially of rice, west of the Wallace line. In addition, rice is good raw material for the preparation of fermented drinks, whose use was unknown in the pre-European period to those Oceanians, tuber cultivators, who lived east of this line.

But all of this cannot explain such a drastic change as the passage from production of starchy perennial plants to cultivation of cereals. Besides, rice seems to have originated in the humid tropics of Indo-Malaysia (Chatterjee, 1951; Burkill, 1953; Richharia, 1960; Barrau, 1965) and it is difficult to imagine that the gardeners of olden times would abandon their starchy perennials in order to domesticate what was probably merely a weed in the taro beds (Haudricourt, 1962).

On the other hand, it is conceivable that immigrants from Asia, accustomed to cultivating and using cereal (the millet *Setaria* perhaps?), came once to Indo-Malaysia, established themselves as conquerers, and cultivated their usual cereal; but they found rice there, so they domesticated it, then spread or enforced its cultivation at the expense of previously dominant perennial food planters.

One might object that this is pure speculation; this is true, and we are here straying from the methods belonging to the natural sciences. But, as De Candolle (1912:6) wrote so well in his *Origine des plantes cultivees:* "The naturalist here is no longer in his usual area of observations and descriptions." Why is he forbidden to use his imagination? Archaeological research will confirm or deny the hypothesis.

This sketch of the food system of Oceania and of what may have been its history will now permit us to bring out some other characteristics of its nutritional ethnobotany.

Plant food is everywhere the dominant part of the diet, and everywhere the starchy plants, grains, tubers, and fruits are the basic foods, making up, as mentioned earlier, as much as 80% and more of the total quantity of foods eaten.

The distinction which certain Melanesians make, for example, those of New Caledonia (Leenhardt, 1937), between *food*—that is, the starchy plant or plants—and *condiments*, comprising various vegetables, meat, fish, etc., embellishing the food diet and enhancing its flavor, seems to be a valid one for the whole of the Malay-Oceanian area; west of the Wallace line, as a general rule, there cannot be a meal without rice; east of this line, a person is considered unfed unless the menu includes either sago, taro, yam, banana, breadfruit, or sweet potato.

The species which are traditionally cultivated or used as the *food,* in other words the *basic food plants,* are few in number. As an example, if we consider Oceania in the strict sense of the term, meaning the New Guinea-Melanesia-Micronesia-Polynesia group, we find only the following plants in this category:

(a) the sago-palms of the genus *Metroxylon.*

(b) members of the Araceae with nourishing tubers, the most important of which are the taro (*Colocasia esculenta* (L.) Schott), *Alocasia macrorrhiza* Schott, *Amorphophallus campanulatus* Blume and *Crytosperma chamissonis* (Schott) Merr.; *Alocasia* and *Amorphophallus* are mentioned here just to recall their existence, since the former has remained important in only a few places, for example in central Polynesia, while the latter has dropped out of use.

(c) members of the Dioscoreaceae, or yams, of the following species: *Dioscorea alata* L., *D. bulbifera* L., *D. esculenta* (Lour.) Burk., *D. hispida* Dennst., *D. nummularia* Lamk., and *D. pentaphylla* L., of which the first, third, and fifth are the most important.

(d) the bananas of the Eumusa group related to *Musa acuminata* Colla and *M. balbisiana* Colla (formerly *Musa paradisiaca* L. and *M. sapientum* L.), and the one from the Australimusa group, *Musa troglodytarum* L., or *fehi.*

(e) a member of the Moraceae, the breadfruit, *Artocarpus altilis* (Park.) Fosb.

(f) finally, a member of the Convolvulaceae, the sweet potato, *Ipomoea batatas* (L.) Lamk., discussed earlier.

Of these plants, the ones that are cultivated are multiplied by vegetative means and are represented by a large variety of clones. Those of the taro, *Colocasia,* and of the major yams, especially those of *Dioscorea alata* L. or large yam, are still not well enough known and a thorough study of the variation of these important cultigens remains to be done; this is also true of the breadfruit. It must be emphasized that these cultigens were and still are almost completely unknown to tropical agronomical science which, as noted previously, is more interested in the cereals and commercial cultivation! This same agronomical science has demonstrated for a long time the same disdain and the same lack of understanding for the traditional horticultural techniques used in the production of these plants. Generalized criticisms, hasty and poorly founded, made so often by colonial agronomists and foresters about food gardening with long-term forested fallow cycles—mistakenly considered a devastating and little productive "shifting cultivation"—were typical of this attitude. Besides its effectiveness in maintaining the delicate fertility of tropical soils, this system has unquestionable advantages in sanitation. Thus, all attempts at cultivation of the taro or the large yam in monoclonal fields result in the rapid appearance of diseases which are often latent in the traditional gardens, but which then take on an increased virulence; at such a moment one finds out that little or nothing is known about them! The above is mentioned simply to demonstrate that there is long overdue a study devoted to these starchy perennial plants which, in tropical Oceania, just as in other parts of the humid tropics, play a basic role in the life of the men living in these regions.

At this point, something should be said about the introduced food plants, in order to bring out a piece of evidence that might well be emphasized. The Oceanian gardeners who cultivated and ate the starchy perennial plants just mentioned accepted without too much difficulty those introduced food plants which resembled or were comparable to the ones they were accustomed to. This explains, for instance, the swift adoption of the *yautia* or *Xanthosoma sagittifolium* (L.) Schott., of the Araceae family, as well as the manioc, *Manihot esculenta* Crantz, two cultigens that were introduced from the American tropics into the islands of the Pacific during the last century; this also explains the success that the sweet potato had when it arrived during the colonial period in those parts of Oceania where it was still unknown. The same could be said of a more recent case, the adoption of another tuber of American origin, the potato, by the Melanesians of the Loyalty Islands in the New Caledonian archipelago. On the other hand, attempts to develop the cultivation of rice, as noticed earlier, always or nearly always failed in the indigenous communities of the lands east of the Wallace line.

As for the *complementary food plants,* those which provide the *condiment,* as distinguished above, their numbers are vast. The inventory of these plants has been attempted elsewhere (Massal and Barrau, 1956; Barrau, 1962) and the reader is referred to it. In order not to burden this essay with details, I will settle here for a general treatment of them. First, one point should be made: although certain of these complementary food plants are cultivated, a large number of them are obtained by wild harvesting. This is especially so in the Melanesian islands and in New Guinea; Blackwood (1940), in his list of the food plant complex of the Kukukukus living in the

New Guinea mountains, noted the use of 52 wild food species! It is a fact that in tropical Oceania gathering of wild plants and cultivation often coexist.

Of food plants that are harvested in the wild state, special mention should be made of those which provide edible seeds, because they play an important part in the dietary balance and because the discussion so far has been limited mainly to the starchy perennials, particularly the tubers. Ames (1939) quite rightly emphasized the great role played by angiosperm seeds in the history of human civilizations, but it should perhaps be remembered that pteridophytes and gymnosperms contributed and continue to contribute considerably to man's nourishment: *Cycas* ovules still are eaten in certain islands of Oceania despite their toxicity, which is removed through skillful methods of preparation; the seeds of *Agathis* and *Auraucaria* were also in demand. It is true, however, that the use of angiosperm seeds is, or at least was, more common. In some places, certain seeds have a definite economic importance; this is the case of certain *Pandanus* plants from the mountains of New Guinea where a species such as *P. jiulianettii* Mart. is exploited through gathering in the wild state as well as being subject to a sort of cultivation. Also in New Guinea, edible seeds are furnished as well by some species which might be worth domesticating and improving; for example, *Terminalia kaernbachii* Warb., (Combretaceae), also *Finschia chloroxantha* Diels (Proteaceae), found as far as southern New Hebrides and used in a large area of Melanesia, as are *Canarium indicum* L. (Burseraceae) and *Barringtonia edulis* Seem. (Lecythidaceae). Several of these species have a somewhat special status intermediate between the wild and domesticated states, in that man protects them in varying degrees by encouraging their reproduction, sheltering them, or helping them. The Polynesian chestnut, *Inocarpus fagiferus* (Park.) Fosberg, a member of the Leguminosae, is also such a case; it is of Indo-Malayan origins and is found and used from the Philippines to eastern Polynesia. While on the topic of plants with edible seeds, we might remember that the breadfruit, in its wild forms, is sought more for its seeds than for its fruit. It is even imaginable that these were the seeds that the navigators of old carried into the islands of the East Pacific where, from among the descendants of the plants thus grown, they chose the seedless clones commonly cultivated today.

It is with a purpose that I dwell here on the complementary food plants that are exploited by gathering in their natural habitat, although sometimes protected by the men who use their products; such protection may go almost as far as cultivation through the arrangement of settlements and human help in propagating these species. Belonging in this category of complementary food plants gathered wild are some that are often labeled "famine foods" or "foods of want." The name is justified by the fact that they are sometimes used in the gaps between harvests of the main food crops or when these crops have failed or have been destroyed by some disaster. Thus, one reads that *Cycas rumphii* Miq. or *Pueraria lobata* (Wild.) Ohwi are "famine food" plants. This seems to me to be a rather hasty interpretation of their true status. Several of these species appear, in fact, to be basic food plants of times past, whose use is still known when the need arises. Far from being treated with disdain, they are truly often a source of prestigious or quasi-ritual foods. This is so of the two species just cited and numerous others which could be given as examples besides. The *Pueraria* referred to above was still cultivated in New Caledonia during the last century; it has disappeared from gardens and today is harvested in the "bush"; its tuber, however, is still considered a choice dish in certain parts of the island. Such plants deserve the attention of ethnobotanists, if only because of their informative value concerning the former use of food plants that were once the basis of subsistence economy.

Among the complementary food plants are found also some species with multiple uses, of which the best example is probably the coconut palm, *Cocos nucifera* L. This providential palm supplies food, drink, fiber, construction and basket-making materials, natural utensils, etc. Another many-sided plant is *Gnetum gnemon* L. (Gnetaceae) which produces edible fruit and leaves and provides a fiber that is especially sought in the making of fish lines and nets, as well as for bowstrings.

For a complete picture, many other species would have to be mentioned, of which some cultivated ones are characteristic of the region. Such is *Hibiscus Manihot* L., which is propagated by cuttings and is very diversified; its leaves make a much valued vegetable in the Sunda Islands as well as in Melanesia, as is also true of the unripened inflorescence of *Saccharum edule* Hassk.

Certain complementary food plants of the Malay-Oceania area took on a new economic importance during the colonial period; the coconut is an example of such food plants that became cultivated for commercial purposes; another is sugar cane which, it is to be remembered, originated in New Guinea.

The few examples mentioned have already shown something of the diversity of complementary plant foods to which the inhabitants of Oceania had, and still have, access. They allow embellishment of the basically starchy diet and assure the completeness of its nutritive value.

From a nutritional point of view, the Oceanian diet has often been wrongly judged, because it had too large a proportion of starchy foods. Probably this was a hasty conclusion based upon the use of questionable criteria: there has always been too great a tendency in this field to take as a model the food that is typical of the European civilizations! What seems clear is that we have too often underestimated both the nutritive contribution of the very numerous complementary food plants that are often eaten between the main meals, thus being missed by the researcher, as well as the nourishment value of certain starchy plants, such as the taro or the yams.

To mention only New Guinea and the islands of Melanesia, Micronesia, and Polynesia, it can be said that malnutrition as a general rule is and was unknown so long as the islanders kept to their traditional foods. The only serious problems of alimentation arising are those of infant nutrition at the point of late and brutal weaning, and those caused by protein deficiencies in some areas of the New Guinea mountains where the water fauna is scarce and where hunting is as poorly productive as the minor raising of stock, particularly pigs.

In fact, problems most often arise when the customary diet is abandoned, because the indigenous people do not know how to use the imported foods or no longer have access to the complementary foods of their usual diet. This is the case of most of the populations that have been urbanized or are being urbanized.

Briefly, east of the Wallace line during the pre-colonial period, the food economy based upon the use of starchy perennial plants gave man good nourishment while there was peace and while no calamity prevented or impeded activities involving food. Today, new economic and social conditions are being set up. Just one example of this is the development of commercial cultivation techniques which compete with food supply activities. However, this is not the most serious aspect of the situation. Before now, there has not often been any imbalance between population and resources. The same cannot be said today; in some islands, notably in the small Polynesian islands, annual rates of population growth as high as 4% have been noted. Already in some places the fallow periods must be shortened for lack of land and this can only result in a dangerous impoverishment of the soils. Already, some introduced food plants such as manioc are increasing in importance even though they are inferior in quality to the traditional plant foods, but they are easier to produce and require less care. Of course, it should be possible to maintain the importance of traditional food cultivars which could be made marketable. To do this would require the modernization of methods of cultivation, the protection of crops from pests and diseases, and the genetic improvement of the plants taking into account their new production conditions . . . but to do this would involve a better knowledge of these plants in which agronomy has taken so little interest to date.

Cultural difficulties also block the way; the Melanesian horticulturist of New Caledonia will refuse to offer for sale some noble yam or taro clone, because it is reserved for ceremonial exchanges only or else it is imbued with such symbolic value that it would be sacrilege to commercialize it. These plants formed an integral part of a system of food economics wherein man sought prestige and not profit and where he held for the plants that he cultivated the respectful friendship that Haudricourt (1964) found important.

The subsistence horticulture of former times was part of the basis of social life. This explains its persistence to this day, but it also explains the problems that the Oceanian societies have in adjusting to a modern monetary economy. These difficulties will have, and are having already, consequences in the area of nutrition. Without underestimating the complexity of the task ahead, we can see that ethnobotany could find here an opportunity for practical application, it could aid in the required evolution by facilitating communication between agronomists and the indigenous farmers; such communication until now has been practically nonexistent in the domain of food horticulture.

Besides, who knows but what certain food plants of the Oceanians might be able to contribute substantially to the solution of that agonizing hunger problem known to so many tropical regions?

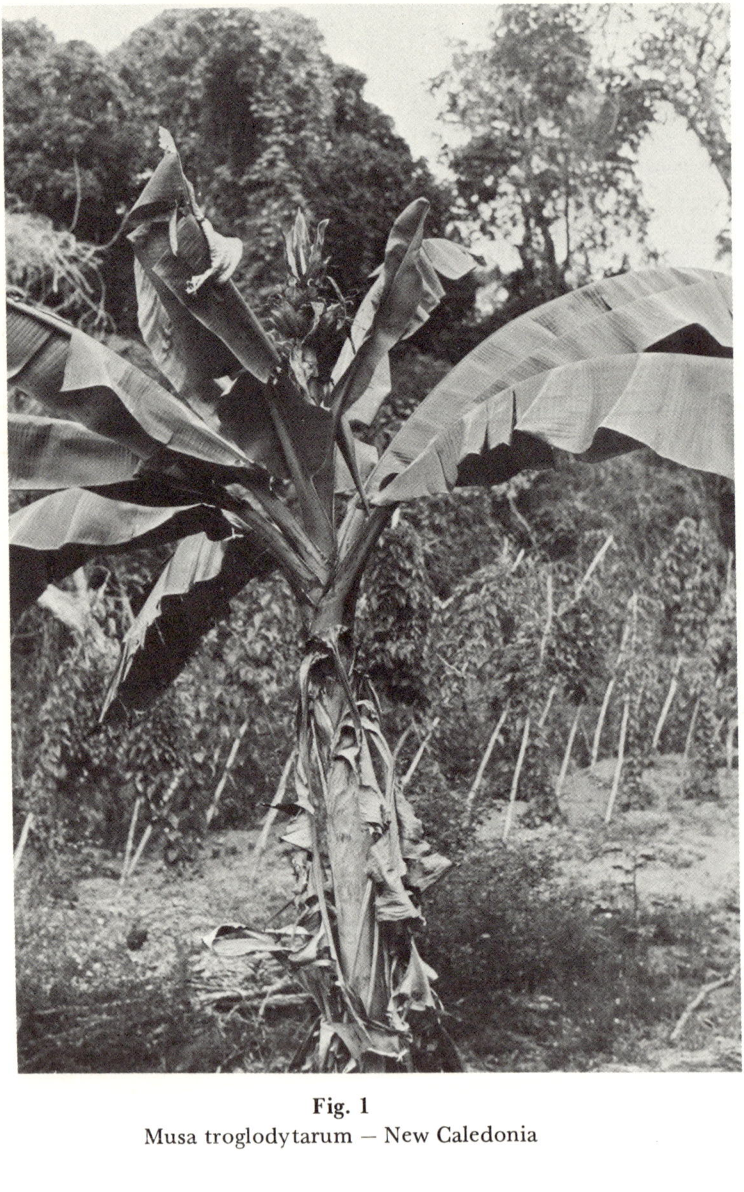

Fig. 1

Musa troglodytarum – New Caledonia

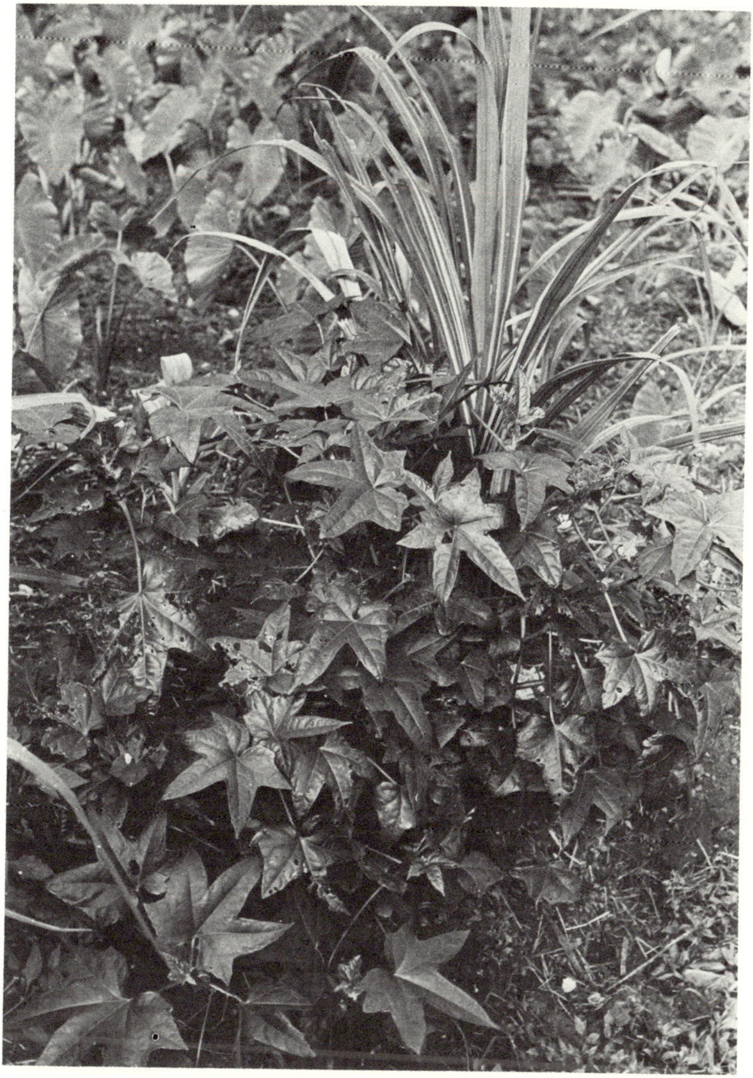

Fig. 2

Hibiscus manihot – a Malayo-Oceanian Vegetable – New Caledonia

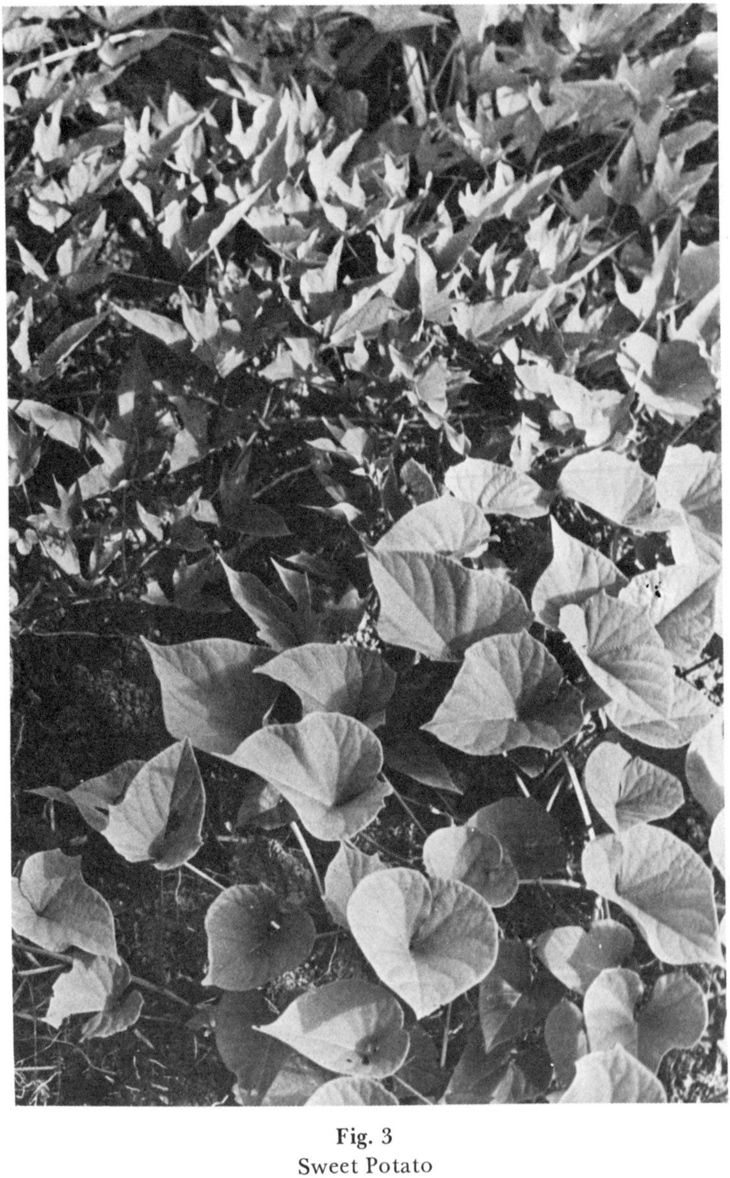

Fig. 3
Sweet Potato

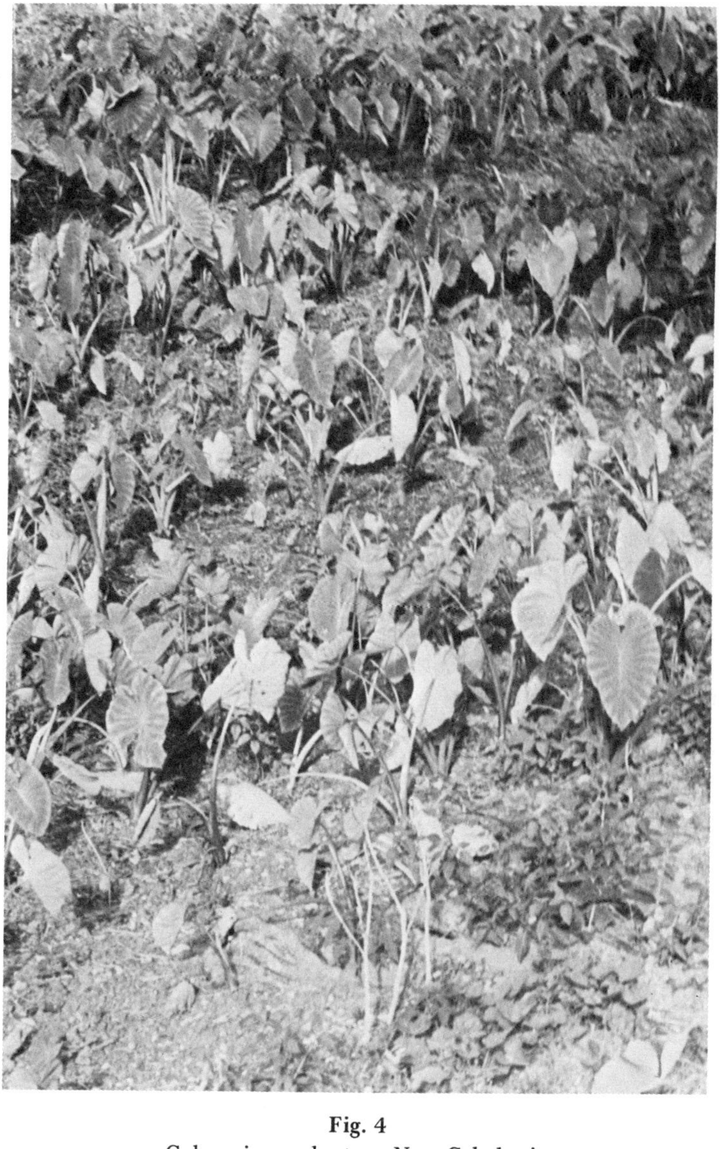

Fig. 4
Colocasia esculenta – New Caledonia

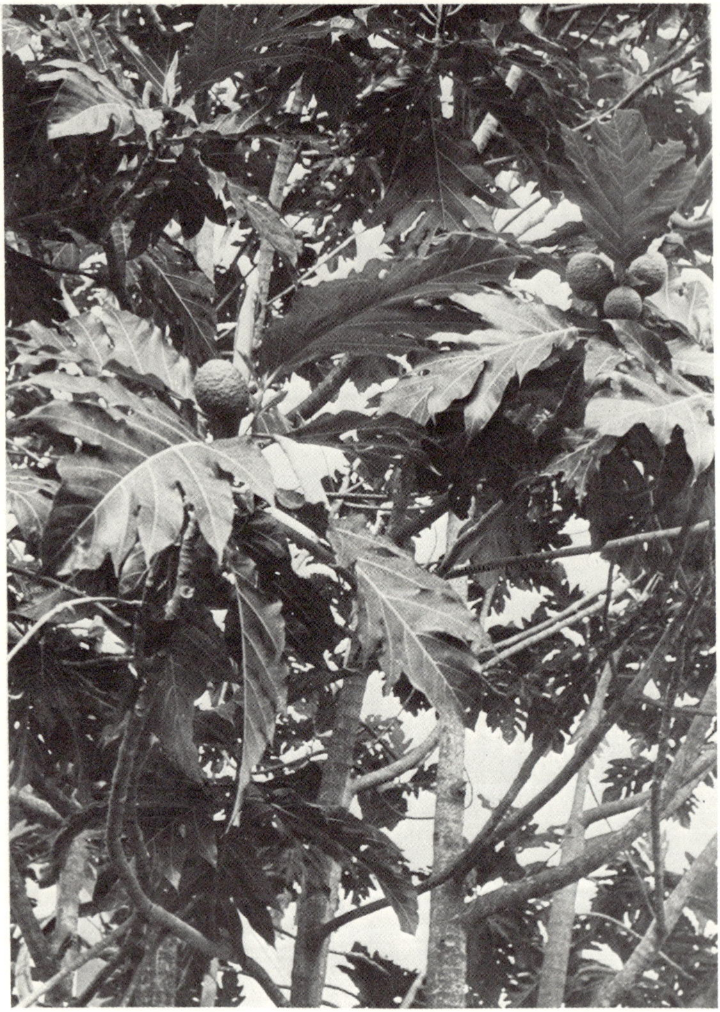

Fig. 5
Artocarpus altilis – The Breadfruit Tree – New Caledonia

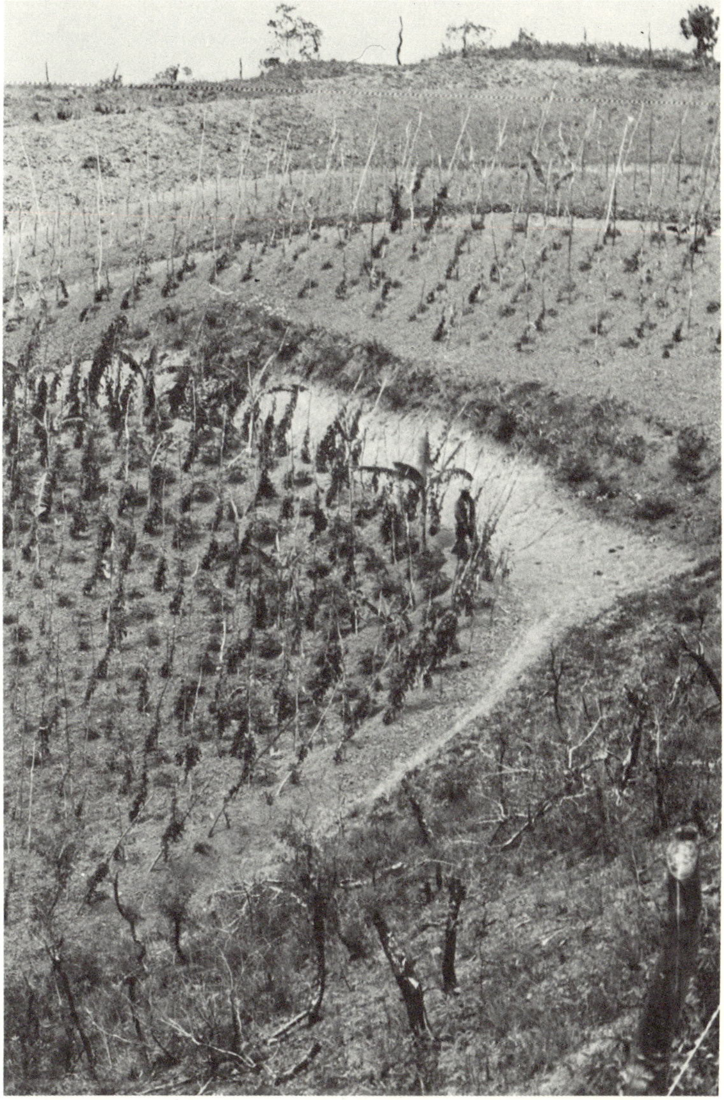

Fig. 6
A Yam Garden – New Caledonia

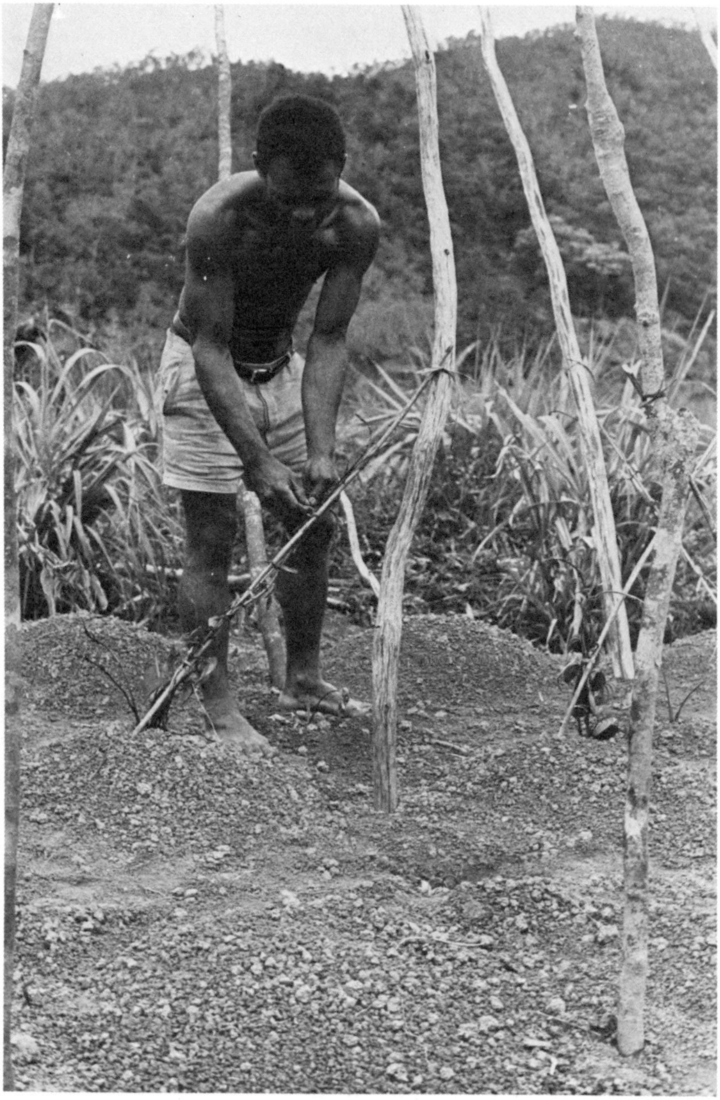

Fig. 7

Melanesian Taking Care of Growing Yam – New Caledonia

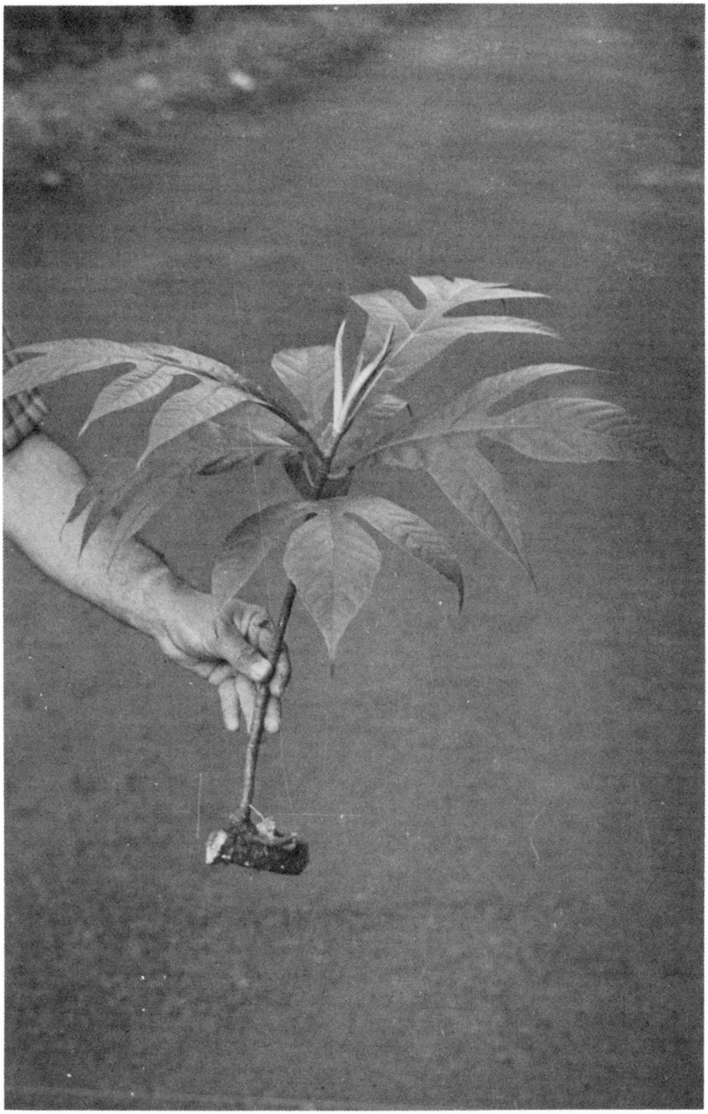

Fig. 8
Breadfruit Root Cutting – Tahiti

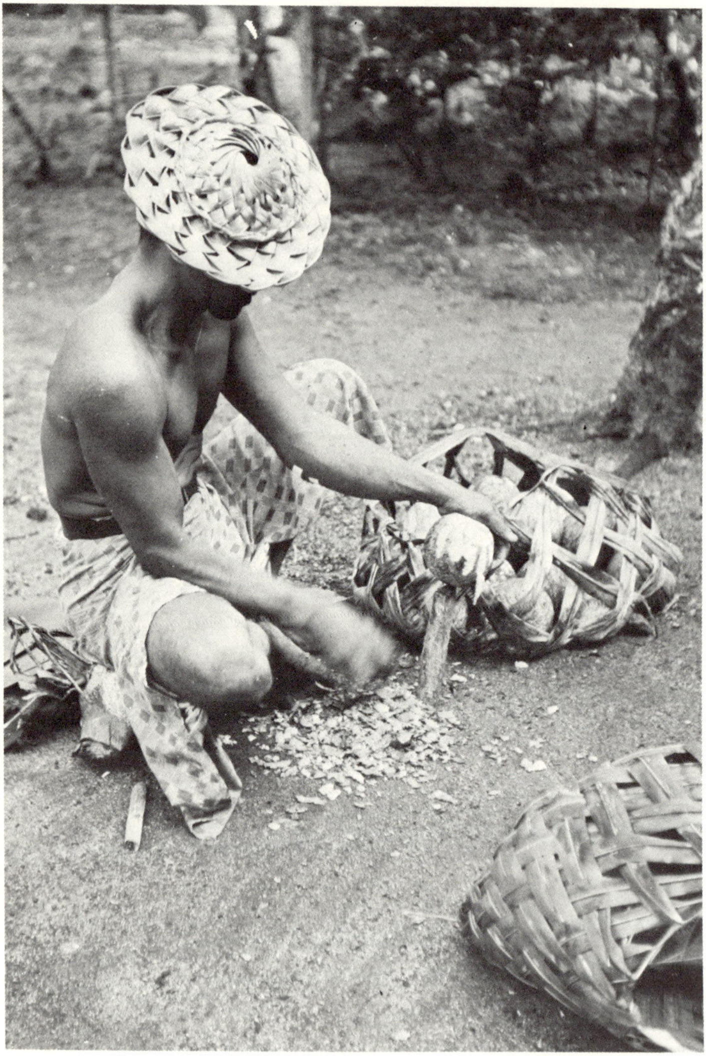

Fig. 9
Scraping the Breadfruit – Manua Island – Eastern Samoa

REFERENCES

Ames, O., 1939. *Economic annuals and human culture,* Botanical Museum Harvard University, Cambridge, Mass.

Artschwager, E., and Brandes, E. W., 1958. *Sugar Cane (Saccharum officinarum* L.) *origin, classification, characteristics, and description of representative clones;* Agriculture handbook 122; U.S. Department of Agriculture, Washington.

Barrau, J., 1959. "Le fabuleux arbre à pain," *Naturalia,* 69: 7-13, Paris.

———, 1962. *Les plantes alimentaires de l'Océanie, origines, distribution et usages* (Annales du Musée Colonial de Marseille, 7e série, vol. 3 à 9), Faculté des Sciences, Marseille.

———, 1965. "L'Humide et le Sec, an essay on ethnobiological adaptation to contrastive environments in the Indo-Pacific," *The Journal of the Polynesian Society,* 74. 3: 329-346, Wellington.

———, 1965. "Witnesses of the Past: Notes on Some Food Plants of Oceania," *Ethnology,* 4. 3: 282-294, Pittsburgh.

———, 1965. "Histoire et préhistoire horticole de l'Océanie tropicale," *Journal de la Société des Océanistes,* 21. 21: 55-78, Paris.

———, 1966. *An ethnobotanical guide for antropological research in Malayo-Oceania* (preliminary draft), mimeo, UNESCO Science Cooperation Office for South East Asia, Bangkok-Djakarta.

———, 1967. "De l'homme cueilleur à l'homme cultivateur," *Cahiers d'Histoire Mondiale,* X. 2: 275-292, Neuchatel.

Blackwood, B., 1940. "Use of plants among the Kukukuku of South Eastern Central New Guinea," *Proceedings of the sixth Pacific Science Congress,* 6: 111-134, University of California Press, Berkeley and Los Angeles.

Burkill, I. H., 1953. "Habits of Man and the Origin of Cultivated Plants of the Old World," *Proceedings of the Linnean Society of London,* 164° session, 1: 12-41, London.

Candolle, A. de, 1912. *L'Origine des plantes cultivées,* revised edition of the version of 1882), Paris.

Chang, K. C., 1968. "Ancient Farmers in the Asian Tropics: Major Problems for Archeological and Palaeoenvironmental Investigations of South-East Asia at the Earliest Neolithic Level" (manuscript, 23 pp., mimeo., kindly made available by the author and to be included in the miscellany in honor of D. Sen, the University of Calcutta).

Chatlerjee, D., 1951. "Notes on the Origin and Distribution of Wild and Cultivated Rices," *Indian Journal of Genetics and Plant Breeding,* special number: symposium on the origin and distribution of cultivated plants in Eastern Asia, 11. 1: 18-22.

Conklin, H. C., 1963. "The Oceanian-African Hypothesis and the Sweet Potato," *Plants and the migration of Pacific peoples* (published under the direction of J. Barrau), Bishop Museum, Honolulu.

Golson, J., 1968. Beyond the Wallace line: New Guinea, Australia and Island Melanesa (manuscript, 27 pp., mimeo., kindly made available by the author and to be included in *Ancient Chinese Art and its Possible Influence in the Pacific Basin,* under the direction of N. Barnard, Australian National University).

Haudricourt, A. G., 1962. "Domestication des animaux, culture des plantes et civilisation d'autrui," *L'Homme,* 2. 1: 40-50, Paris.

———, 1964. "Nature et culture dans la civilisation de l'igname, origines des clones et des clans," *L'Homme,* 4: 93-104, Paris.

Haudricourt, A. G., and Hédin, L., 1943. *L'Homme et les plantes cultivees,* Paris.

Lathrap, D. W., 1965. "Origin of Central Andean Civilisation: New Evidence," *Science,* 148: 3671.

Leenhardt, M., 1937. *Gens de la Grande Terre,* Paris.

MacDaniels, L. H., 1947. *A Study of the Fe'i Banana and its Distribution in Relation to Polynesian Migrations* (Bernice P. Bishop Museum Bulletin No. 190), Honolulu.

Massal, E., and Barrau, J., 1956. "Food Plants of the South Sea Islands," *South Pacific Commission technical paper* no. 94, Nouméa.

Nishiyama, I., 1963. "The Origin of the Sweet Potato Plant," *Plants and the Migrations of Pacific Peoples* (published under the direction of J. Barrau), Bishop Museum, Honolulu.

Riccharia, R. H., 1960. "Origin of Cultivated Rices," *Indian Journal of Genetics and Plant Breeding,* 20. 1: 1-14.

Sahlins, M., 1968. "La première société d'abondance," *Les temps modernes,* 268, Paris.

Sauer, C. O., 1952. *Agricultural Origins and Dispersals, Bowman Memorial Lectures,* Series 2, American Geographical Society, New York.

Segawa, K., and Kano, T., 1956. *An Illustrated Ethnography of the Formosan Aborigines,* Vol. 1, *the Yami,* Tokyo.

Simmonds, N. W., 1959. *Bananas,* London.

Vavilov, N. I., 1951. *The origin, variation, immunity and breeding of cultivated plants* (collection of selected works translated by Starr Chester, Waltham).

Warner, J. N., 1962. "Sugar Cane, an Indigenous Papuan Cultigen," *Ethnology,* 1. 4: 405-411.

Watson, J. B., 1964. "Anthropology in the New Guinea Highlands," *American Anthropologist,* 66. 4: 2.

Wilder, G. P., 1928. *The Breadfruit in Tahiti* (Bernice P. Bishop Museum Bulletin No. 50) Honolulu.

Yen, D. E., 1963. "Sweet Potato Variation and its Relation to Human Migrations in the Pacific," *Plants and the Migrations of Pacific Peoples* (published under the direction of J. Barrau) Bishop Museum, Honolulu.

Botanical Glossary

Agathis – The pine family (Pinaceae) includes this broad-leaved genus with edible seeds. Perhaps its best known representative is the kauri pine of New Zealand, which is commercially exploited for lumber and gum.

Agave – The many species of *Agave* (family Amaryllidaceae) are used for food (flower buds, leaf bases, and the stem), for fiber (leaves and flower stalk), for beverages, made from the sap, both sweet (agua miel), fermented (pulque), and distilled (tequila, mescal) and for soap (flesh or green fruit). During the dry season in Mexico and the southwestern United States, these plants may have furnished the principal vegetable food prehistorically for people who were food gatherers.

agriculture – Technically, the cultivation of plants in fields (from *agri* – Latin, *ager,* field) which seems to have developed in the Old World with the use of draft animals. In the New World, the lack of draft animals precluded the development of agriculture in the same form, but extensive hand-cultivated fields must have been made to supply the quantities of tribute recorded in documents of the Conquest era.

Amaranthus – Probably best known as pigweed, this genus of the Amaranthaceae has long been cultivated in the Americas for its seed. The leaves are also edible as greens. In Mexico at the present time, the seeds are popped and mixed with honey to make *alegria,* a confection commonly sold on the streets.

Artocarpus – A genus of the Moraceae or fig family. The widely cultivated breadfruit is primarily esteemed in the Pacific area, where it is known in many cultivated varieties.

Arctostaphylos – This genus of the Ericaceae (blueberry family), includes shrubs and trees in western and northern North America. Included are the manzanitas of California whose berries were widely used, but at least one Mexican species is reported to have a narcotic principle in the fruit, which has poisoned children. Other species are used medicinally.

Auraucaria – Confined solely to the southern hemisphere, this genus of the pine family (Pinaceae) is known primarily by the decorative Norfolk Island pine. Seeds of the species of the genus were gathered and used as food both in South America and in the Old World. Many of the tree trunks in Petrified Forest of Arizona are auraucarian fossils.

Barringtonia – The Brazil nut family (Lecythidaceae) is more widely known for the commercially available Brazil and paradise nuts from South America than it is for the edible-seeded species of the Old World.

beans – Any of a number of seeds of plants in the bean family (Leguminosae), although the name is applied most frequently to the common bean (*Phaseolus vulgaris*). Fully ripe lima beans (*P. lunatus*) are high in starch, but most are high in protein. Common and lima beans were domesticated in the Americas by at least 5,000 BC in both Mexico and Peru.

breadfruit – The large fruit of a tropical tree of the mulberry or fig family (Moraceae) is used in many tropical areas, although it apparently originated in Indo-Malaya. Perhaps it was originally collected from the wild for its nutritious seeds, but domestication led to the development of seedless varieties whose flesh is highly valued.

Canarium – Although this genus has a few members whose seeds are considered edible, other members of the genus and the family Burseraceae are widely exploited for their fragrant resins such as the copals of Mexico and myrrh in southwestern Asia and Northern Africa.

Capsicum – This genus includes the chili peppers, used for flavoring and sauces, and the sweet bell peppers, used for cooking and salads. It is a member of the potato family (Solanaceae). It has been used since at least 7,000 BC (Tehuacan Valley plant remains) and it has been widely distributed around the world only since the Spanish Conquest of Mexico.

Ceiba – A genus of the silk cotton family (Bombacaceae), the *Ceiba* tree of the American tropics has often been held to be sacred. It is often an obvious giant even in a forest of 120-foot tall trees. *C.*

pentandra is a source of kapok fiber (used for packing of pillows and life jackets etc., but too smooth to spin) while *C. parvifolia* of the Tehuacan Valley is valued for its edible seeds and large storage roots as well.

chili – The fruit of the pepper plant (*Capsicum annuum,* usually), widely used in Mexican cuisine. Although frequently used as a spice in the preparation of other foods, a sauce made of freshly chopped chilis, husk tomatoes, vinegar, etc., is served almost daily in some parts of Mexico.

Cocos – The genus to which the coconut belongs is a member of the palm family (Palmae). Long conceded to be one of the world's most useful plants, coconuts are commercially exploited for oil and fiber. Locally, they furnish food, kitchen utensils, string, rope, matting, basketry, roofing, structural members for building, and other items. The coconut was apparently brought into cultivation in the Old World, but the number of its relatives in the New World has led to assumptions that it originated in the Americas.

Coix – This genus of the grass family (Gramineae) originated in the Old World, but it is now widely distributed. The hard, gray fruits are used as food in the Philippines, but in other parts of the world they are used principally as beads.

Colocasia – A member of the arum family (Araceae), this genus includes the taro, which is an important carbohydrate source for people of the Indo-Pacific area. As long as the roots are not dug, they remain firm and good to use. Thus, a taro patch can be successively harvested over a period of time, precluding loss during storage. In some parts of the area of its growth, storage is impossible because of high rainfall and humidity.

Cordyline – Species of this genus of the lily family (Liliaceae) are often called ti in the South Pacific area, where the enlarged storage roots are roasted and eaten or prepared into a beverage. The roots have a high sugar content and licorice flavor. Many varieties were once cultivated, primarily in Melanesia, but *Cordyline* has not become popular in other parts of the world.

Cucurbita – The New World genus of five cultivated species which include the squashes, pumpkins, and marrows. *C. pepo, C. moschata,* and *C. mixta* apparently originated in Mexico or Central America, the first being in cultivation from about 7,000 BC (Oaxaca caves). *C. maxima* was brought into cultivation in South America and *C. ficifolia* probably came into cultivation in Central America.

Cycas – An Old World genus of the ancient family Cycadaceae (the cycad family is known from fossils 350 million years old), the seeds of *Cycas* have been used as food. However they contain a chemical which causes damage to nerve tissue, particularly if improperly prepared.

Dioscorea – A genus of the yam family (Dioscoreaceae). Yam cultivation is apparently a very old form of plant husbandry.

Diospyros – A genus of the ebony family (Ebenaceae) which produces fruit known as Sapote negro in Mexico and persimmon in the United States. The fruits obviously were highly regarded prehistorically, because remains have been found in the Tehuacan caves which date to as early as 4,800 BC.

Empetrum – Widely used around the Northern hemisphere, *E. nigrum* of the crowberry family (Empetraceae) has long provided some of the dietary elements lacking in a diet largely confined to storable vegetable products and animal protein during the winter months. The insipid berries were dried or pounded into meat for storage.

Finschia – A small genus of the family Proteaceae, it is little known outside of its native area. The most widely known member of this family is the tree producing macadamia nuts.

Hibiscus – Many plants belonging to the mallow family (Malvaceae) have fibrous layers in the stem which have been widely used. *H. tiliaceus* is exploited also for an edible inner bark, although it is more frequently planted today throughout the tropics as an ornamental tree, particularly along streets and close to salt water.

Inocarpus – Another member of the bean family (Leguminosae) whose seeds are utilized. Like many plant families producing popular foods, the bean family includes some poisonous members such as the Malabar or ordeal beans of Africa.

Ipomoea – A genus of the morning-glory family (Convolulaceae) to which the sweet potato belongs. This plant was apparently brought into cultivation in the Caribbean region. Many varieties are known which are maintained in tropical agriculture by means of vegetative propagation like most crops originating and used in the wet tropics around the world.

Lemaireocereus – The species of this genus of the cactus family (Cactaceae) are mostly large arboreal cacti. Fruit of most of the species is edible and the stem tissue of some is edible. The large spines of *L. weberi* were used prehistorically as pins. Fruit of most of the species in southern Mexico ripens in April at the end of the long dry season marking the end of a period of monotonous diet.

lichen – A symbiotic array of an alga and a fungus. While the alga or fungus may be cultured separately, when they grow together, they form an identifiable organism in which neither one nor the other component is dominant. The kind referred to here is often called "reindeer moss," but other prominent kinds are rock tripe, grandad's beard, and British soldiers. In much of the temperate zone, the most conspicuous kinds are the grey-green to yellow-green species adhering closely to rocks and tree trunks.

Maize (corn) – The seed of a species of the genus *Zea* which is a grass. Because of its productivity, maize is an important grain for human and domesticated animal consumption at the present time. However, remains of early maize from ca. 5,000 BC in the Tehuacan Valley indicate that these plants were not nearly so productive and the plant may have been more highly valued for the sugar content of its stems.

mesquite – Trees of the genus *Prosopis* of the bean family, leguminosae, whose pods and seeds are used in western North America and South America (where it is known as algaroba). Material around the seeds is sweet and can be boiled down in water to make syrup. The seeds can be ground and are highly proteinaceous.

Metroxylon – A genus of the palm family (Palmae) which includes the sago palm. Much sago starch is locally gathered from the center of the trunks of wild trees, but some plantations produce commercial sago starch and a hard, granular product known as pearl sago.

Musa – The genus of the banana belonging to the Musaceae or banana family. Bananas originated in the Old World as a hybrid of two wild species. Cultivated varieties of bananas and plantains are completely sterile and must be increased by planting parts of an underground stem or rhizome. Varieties include many hundreds of sweet or dessert bananas and starchy cooking plantains.

Opuntia – The genus of the cactus family (Cactaceae) to which the prickly pear and cholla cacti belong. Often the fruit and the stems, "pads," are edible. Blockage of the intestines has been reported to have been caused by ingestion of too many fruit at one time, because they are largely seeds with only a small amount of flesh.

Oryza – A genus of the grass family (Gramineae) which includes *Oryza sativa,* cultivated rice. This crop originated either in India or southeast Asia, perhaps at an early time. Archaeological remains from India are dated ca. 2,000 BC.

Oxyria – This genus of the Polygonaceae has a distribution primarily in the Arctic. *O. digyna* has long been used as a source of greens among the Eskimos and the Indians.

Oxytropus – A widely distributed genus of the Leguminosae or bean family in western and northern North America, *Oxytropus* is known locally as locoweed, because the tops of the plants poison grazing animals. Thus, anyone who wishes to duplicate native plant use should accurately identify the plants whose roots they wish to eat.

Pedicularis – A genus of the figwort family (Scrophulariaceae), it includes a common eastern North American woodland species which is locally called lousewort.

platano – The Spanish word for either the dessert banana or the starchy cooking plantain. These probably originated in southeastern Asia, but they were adopted by the forest agriculturists of the American tropics as a major food source. Although vegetatively propagated, many varieties are known.

Polygonum – Belonging to the family Polygonaceae, *Polygonum* is closely related to buckwheat. Several species of the genus are used as potherbs or the roots are used.

Prosopis – A genus of the bean family (Leguminosae), the pods of which are used in both the New World and the Old World for food. Native women in Mexico can still be seen gathering screwbeans or mesquite. It grows principally in drainage areas of dry country where the roots can reach water.

Pueraria – Many plants of the bean family (Leguminosae) have been gathered and subsequently brought into cultivation for their fleshy roots rather than for their seeds or fruits. This Old World genus related to soy beans has several species, including the infamous kudzu vine of the southeastern United States, which fall into this category.

rice – The basic or primary carbohydrate for a large part of the world's population, rice is grown in an upland form and a paddy or irrigated form. The yield from the latter kind of rice is greater, but the labor needed for successful production is also greater.

root – In the strictest botanical sense, this applies only to the portion of the seed bearing plant which provides anchorage and, in the soil, participates in the uptake of material from the soil solution. In culinary use, this may refer to any underground portion of a plant.

Rubus – The blackberries and raspberries of commerce are well known members of this genus. Fruit of all wild members is usable, but some species bear fruit with large seeds and dry flesh, which is unpalatable. The rose family, Rosaceae, to which this belongs, is noted for edible fruits like apple, peach, strawberry, and others.

Rumex – A genus of the knotweed family (Polygonaceae) whose species are often called dock. One species (*R. hymenosepala*) is commercially exploited for the tannic acid content of its roots (canaigre or tanner's dock). Many species of *Rumex* are considered weeds in the temperate zone, one of the most common of which, *R. acetosella,* has been used as greens.

Saccharum – A genus of the grass family (Gramineae) native to the Old World. Sugar cane is a species of this genus. Sources of sugar are often limited, but highly desired. Thus, early discovery and cultivation led to widespread use prehistorically.

sago palm – One of the species of the genus *Metroxylon* in the palm family (Palmae), the sago palm has long been harvested from wild stands for the starch which can be extracted from the trunk. Just prior to blooming, much starch is stored, but it can be obtained only by felling the tree.

Salix – The genus includes many species ranging from large trees to small shrubs. In addition to their value as food, willow shoots are frequently used as material for basketry or mats and the slipped bark can be made into willow whistles or flutes.

screw pine – Not really pines, members of the genus *Pandamus* (Pandanaceae) are widely planted in the tropics as ornamentals. Primarily in the Pacific area where they originated, the seeds and the fruits have been gathered for food. The terminal bud or "heart" where the new leaves are produced is also cooked and eaten.

seed – The ultimate reproductive unit of a seed plant, the seed usually consists of an embryo, with or without a store of nutriment, enclosed in a nearly impermeable coat. It is borne within a fruit except among the cone-bearing plants. Seeds have often been important in human diets because of their high concentrations of oil, proteins, starch or sugars. Some, like wheat, are the principal carbohydrate foods for a large part of the world's population.

Setaria – This genus of the grass family (Gramineae) includes the foxtail millets domesticated in the Old World and *S. macro-*

stachya which apparently was a principal grain of Mexico prior to the domestication and improvement of maize. Some question still remains as to whether *S. macrostachya* was cultivated.

squash — Fruit of any of several native American species of *Cucurbita,* the domesticated forms of which are widely used for human and animal food. Perhaps the wild forbears were collected for their seeds (edible when roasted) and for the highly soapy inedible flesh which is still sometimes used for washing in Mexico. Seeds of cultivated *C. pepo* have been recovered from an Oaxaca cave at a level dated 7,000 BC.

stems — The upper axial portions of seed plants, usually bearing leaves and often flowers and fruits. Stems may be very small, i. e. the button at the base from which grow the fleshy layers of the onion bulb, or large, i. e. the trunk of a tree and its limbs. Most cacti are all stem and no leaves.

sugar cane — A large grass of the genus *Saccharum,* widely cultivated for the sweet juice of its stem. It has been suggested that the wild grass was originally sought for its edible seeds, but this is unlikely in the wet tropical climate of New Guinea, where this plant is a native. Tuberous starch sources are not uncommon, but sources of sugar are rare and seeds are less often produced by a grass that normally reproduces by stem rooting.

sweet potato — A plant of the genus *Ipomoea* which belongs to the morning-glory family (Convolvulaceae). Sweet potato may have been introduced into the Pacific Islands prehistorically from America where it originated. Although it seldom is the primary carbohydrate source in a diet, it is now an important starch food for people and animals throughout the tropics of the world.

taro — Throughout the Pacific area, this underground portion of a species of *Colocasia* (arum family, Araceae) is often the principal carbohydrate source in the diet. Many varieties are known, some of which have restricted uses. An important ritual food, poi, is ground, lightly fermented taro; it has been popularized as a part of Hawaiian luaus.

Terminalia — Many members of this genus are trees, the most prominent of which is *T. catappa,* the tropical almond, whose seed is eaten wherever it is planted throughout the moist tropics.

thorn-scrub — In the western United States and Mexico, often at elevations below 1,800 m where rainfall is less than 600 mm per year concentrated during eight months or less, the arboreal cover for the land is less than 10 m tall, scattered, and frequently spiny. Shrubs in the intervening spaces are often tortuously branched and spiny also. Cacti usually grow in association with this kind of vegetation.

Tillandsia – A genus of the pineapple family (Bromeliaceae), *Tillandsia* species are commonly called air plants, because they cling to the trunks and branches of trees or even utility wires. The most familiar but most aberrant species is Spanish moss. The leaves of many species were once used for their strong fine fiber and some were obviously eaten (see Callen article).

yams – Many species of *Dioscorea,* native to the tropics of both the Old World and the New World, develop edible tubers (storage stems full of starch, which may be borne aerially or underground). Others are inedible because of included chemicals, one of which is the commercially exploited precursor of cortisone. Yams have been domesticated by and are used by lowland forest people in Asia, Africa, and the Americas.

Vaccinium – A genus of the family Ericaceae, of which many species grow throughout eastern and northern North America. Often the berries are edible and delicious. Included are blueberries, cranberries, whortleberries, huckleberries, etc., of which solely the blueberries and the cranberries are cultivated.

Zea – A grass (Gramineae) genus of probably only two species; one, maize or corn, is one of the world's important cereals. It was and is the principal carbohydrate in the diet of native people of Mexico and upland South America. Since the Spanish Conquest, maize has become the principal starch food of the negros of eastern Africa and of some of the people of Asia.

Index